Advanced Praise for

MW01006932

"All of my births became [...] of my children's welcome [...] power, and transformation as a woman becoming a mother. Stories are both information and soul. They are therapy. And they heal both the writer and the listener as we tap into universal human truths and experience. The healing potential of story in birth is profound and only beginning to be tapped into by mothers - mothers who have struggled, lost, succeeded, triumphed and want to make the most of their experience as a journey of growth and being deeply human, deeply woman. **If your journey of birth and motherhood is in need of witness, healing, hearing, or sharing** - and you don't know where to start - or if putting pen to paper makes you freeze up but there's a story that is calling out to be told - *Birth Your Story* **by writer and teacher Jaime Fleres is where I suggest you go to birth your inner writer.**"

AVIVA ROMM
MD, midwife
Author of *The Natural Pregnancy Book* and *Natural Health After Birth*

"Do you know your birth story? And if you are a parent, what do you remember about bringing your own child(ren) into the world? **Jaime Fleres's book, *Birth Your Story*, makes a unique contribution to how we look at birth and why writing our story matters.**

Birth Your Story is part memoir and part writing guide. **I wish I had this book 25 years ago as I was birthing my children.** It would have encouraged me to look at other options for how I wanted to bring a baby into the world. Jaime's book explains what we lose as a culture, as a family and as women when we don't pass on these stories. **This is an important book that will help you discover the gift of creation both in the womb and on the page.**"

BETSY BLANKENBAKER
Author of *Autobiography of an Orgasm*

"No matter what kind of birth experience you had, writing the story is so important for honoring this huge rite of passage. **This book is a meaningful and poignant guide** to telling the story of one of, if not THE, most important experience of your life."

KATE NORTHRUP
Creator of Origin and bestselling author of *Money: A Love Story*

"*Birth Your Story* reads like a midwife or doula feels: **wise, grounded, clear, no bullsh*t, unflappable and totally loving, with a sacred reverence** for the whole wild and winding journey of birth. I personally didn't realize what power there is in writing your birth story, until I wrote my own, and I wonder what secret joy, what humility, and what self-pride, would still be locked inside had I not. What a joy to discover Jaime Fleres' book, that not only guides us through the transformational writing process, but into **a deep reclamation of our body, power, fragility, wisdom and divinity.** Whether a seasoned writer or a blushing novice, no matter: open this book and write on."

LIYANA SILVER
Coach and author of *Feminine Genius: The Provocative Path to Waking Up and Turning On the Wisdom of Being a Woman*

"Jaime Fleres's *Birth Your Story* is the perfect gift for expecting couples and new (and not so new) parents. Jaime's warmth and wisdom encourage and empower readers to begin to write and embrace their birth stories. But this book is so much more than a how-to book; **it's a celebration of love and the power of what our bodies and minds are capable of.** It's a must-have book for any parent in your life."

KATE HOPPER
Author of *Use Your Words: A Writing Guide for Mothers* and *Ready for Air: A Journey Through Premature Motherhood*

"Jaime Fleres guides parents to the pen of self-exploration with kindness, wit, and compassion. Why write our birth stories? Jaime reminds us that in telling our stories, we share our hearts, honor sacred passages, and bring healing insight to both ourselves and our world."

AMY WRIGHT GLENN
Author of *Birth, Breath & Death* and *Holding Space*

"Every woman's story matters. Fleres shares the birth stories of men and women, inspiring readers to embark on the journey of writing their own. The best part is Fleres takes away the intimidation of writing your own story by giving the reader an easy and accessible step-by-step guide to follow."

AMY JOHNSON GRASS
President of the American Association of Birth Centers, founder of
Health Foundations Birth Center, midwife, naturopath

"Every culture has a creation story that is central to its identity, a tale that provides its people with a fundamental understanding of self and our relation to the world. There is no denying the power of these origin stories, just as there is no denying the power and essential importance of a woman's birth story. In telling our birth stories, we reclaim our limitless power as creators, we own our journey as we transition into parenthood, we find agency in our voices and, yes, we add to the collective understanding of the human experience. This beautiful book recognizes and powerfully communicates the vital importance of owning and sharing our birth stories. With great compassion, Jaime clearly communicates not only why telling our stories is so vitally important, but how to tell them in a way that will heal, empower, awaken and enlighten. My greatest wish is that this book inspires you to share your creation story—the beautiful, the heartbreaking, the awe-inspiring and the revolutionary. Your voice matters, your experience counts, and your story takes us all higher."

ELAN VITAL McALLISTER
President and Founder of Choices in Childbirth, producer of *The
Guide to a Healthy Birth*

"Whether a woman has had the birth of her dreams, or the opposite, there is raw ecstasy in fully owning the experience. Jaime Fleres artfully supports women to find their power through writing their stories, sharing not just the details of the birth experience, but exploring their inner landscape in the process. *Birth Your Story* is a heartfelt reminder that in the journey of birthing our babies, we women are being reborn as mothers. Here is a venue to consciously explore and unearth the gifts we've received along the way, alchemizing every drop into showing up more vibrantly as women and mothers."

SHEILA HAYS
Founder of Ecstatic Birth

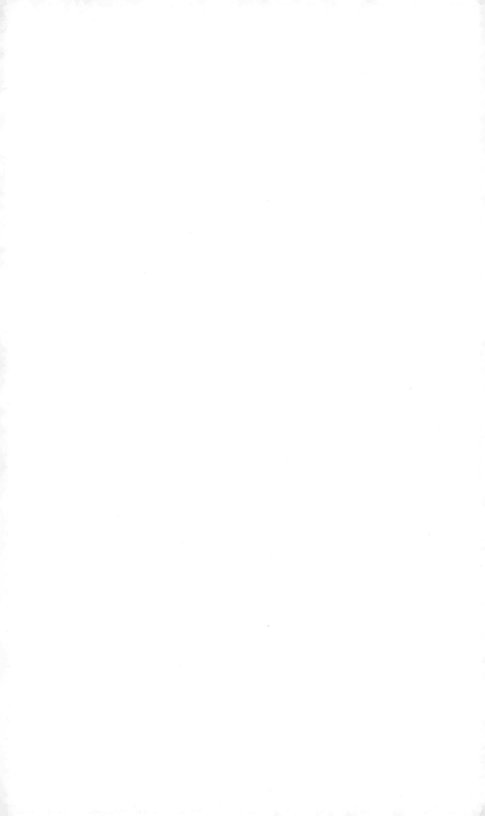

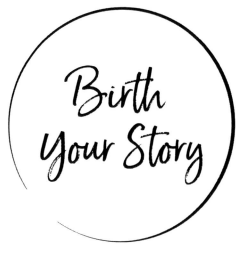

Birth Your Story

Why Writing about Your Birth Matters

Jaime Fleres

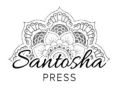

Santosha
PRESS

Editor: Kate Hopper
Copyeditor: Lauren Lang
Proofreader: Amanda Coffin
Design: Emily Bohannon
Cover art: Ana Grigoriu, photo by Danica Donnelly
Author Photo: Sarah Hrudka

For more information about special discounts for bulk purchases, author speaking events and workshops, and more: visit JaimeFleres.com.

Santosha Press
30 Westgate Parkway #339
Asheville, North Carolina 28806

Printed in the United States of America.

ISBN: 978-0-9991637-8-8

DEDICATION

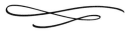

I dedicate this book to my daughter, Maia, the light of my life. Without you, this book surely would not have come through me. You've changed everything in the most delightful of ways, and I am a better person with you in my life.

Lastly, I dedicate this book to women everywhere who ever have or will give birth. You are phenomenal, your stories are important, and you deserve to be heard, supported and cared for—in birth and in all of your days of mothering. It's no easy feat. May you deeply and unshakably know your value, your worth, your beauty, and the sacredness of your love and service.

CONTENTS

(

INTRODUCTION

I've HAD MY SHARE OF ADVENTURES. I've jumped out of planes in California, run right off the edge of mountains in Switzerland, swum through dark caves teeming with screeching bats and cat-sized spiders in Thailand. I've taught squirrel monkeys how to fish. To my knowledge, I was the first ever kettlebell teacher in Peru.

I've twice moved to different countries alone, driven purely by my sense of adventure, and once moved across this country for love. I met my husband in a hot spring under a double rainbow on 11/11 in the Sacred Valley of Peru. We were married by shamans on a Mexican beach three years to the day later.

I've lost a child. I've lost my fertility, my uterus, and my cycles to illness. I've sat beside my father and my father-in-law as they took their last breaths. These losses have broken and remade me stronger.

As rich as this life has been,
nothing has been as wild, as intense,
or as memorable as giving birth.

Absolutely nothing has altered my life as much as bringing my daughter into this world on February 27, 2013.

In the days following Maia's birth, the experience swirled and surged in my mind. Parts of the birth experience would surface, and I'd feel the pull—toward awe, shock, disbelief, gratitude, love, understanding, wow. The mighty need to hold my child—which pierced through every layer of my being—was rivaled only by my fierce desire to process and tell my story of birthing her.

A writer and English professor by trade, I also felt the strong call to write my story down on paper. In fact, it was more than a call: it was a requirement. Putting pen to paper had always been my way of processing and making sense of my experiences. Writing was how I had survived my intensely turbulent teens, early traumas, serial heart-break, and heavy emotions I didn't know what else to do with. Always a trusty guide, writing was essential nourishment after birth.

Between nursing sessions and naps in those early postpartum days, I began writing my story in bed on my laptop. I was driven to capture the details, to make sense of what had happened, to re-member parts of my daughter's birth that were blurry, to discover the truths awaiting me through the writing process (which I knew were not otherwise accessible), and to honor this monumental transforma-tion in my life.

If I hadn't crafted a cohesive narrative, my birth experience would have remained discombobulated fragments of memory that faded with time. Writing my story helped me preserve this cherished memory and come to understand and claim my experience as my own. It also helped me discover the power and meaning behind the birth; it gave me space to recognize and honor the wisdom and sacredness of my body, the feminine, and Life.

In the months following Maia's birth, I was inspired to share this power of expression with other new mamas. As a writer and mother's group facilitator for the birth center where I'd had Maia, I organized a workshop to help others write their birth stories. Present in the work-shop circle were a handful of mothers who'd birthed in the last few years. None of these women considered themselves writers, but all were driven to tell their stories.

Like me, these women yearned to remember, heal, process, and honor their births, their stories, their lives. For the next two hours, we forged authentic connections around our diverse birth experienc-es, readied ourselves for writing with a guided meditation, and had ample time to write. It was so powerful to witness the remembering, the reconnection, the discovery, the love, and the truth these women accessed by opening up to express and write about their births. It felt like such important work. It still does.

Wanting to offer this profound experience to a wider circle, I began writing this book.

Giving birth to Maia was also a time of giving birth to myself. I trained to become a birth doula. I launched a holistic health business to support women in the childbearing season. I privately coached women in their birth-writing journeys. The more I worked with mothers and witnessed their strong need to express their birth experiences, the stronger I felt the pull to develop my initial workshop material into a more substantial book.

While the landscape of literature available to birthing and new parents includes mountains of manuals and streams of story anthologies, what was missing was a book that guided parents in *why* and *how* to write their stories.

My aim in this book is to offer you, as mothers and fathers, a resource to help you understand the value of writing your birth stories as a way of remembering (and recording), processing, claiming, healing, and honoring your birth experiences.

With a philosophy that every birth story
is important and worth telling, this
book is intended to be accessible to all
parents, regardless of their backgrounds,
beliefs, or birth experiences.

This book is divided into three main parts and includes a robust appendix section. In Part One, we explore why writing your birth story matters. Part Two explores the body of our collective and personal birth stories, including our birth story narrative, the three layers of a birth story, and how our stories change through time. In Part Three we journey through the creative process of writing, from start to finish, including how to get started, guidelines for writing, and what to do after you write. The appendices contain many additional resources and exercises that enrich the process of writing birth stories.

Woven throughout the book are birth stories written by men and women across the US. These stories illustrate how rich and varied birth experiences are, and they can be used as models of what birth story-writing can look like. These stories include the voices of an adoptive mother present at the birth of her daughter, a teen father writing seventeen years after his son's birth, and a same-sex couple who brought their son into the world via surrogacy, to name a few. Our storytellers speak of natural birth, medically assisted birth, planned cesarean birth, traumatic birth, and ecstatic birth. Our storytellers are those who recently birthed and those who birthed decades ago; professional writers and those who do not consider themselves writers at all. While our collection doesn't represent all birthing voices, my intention here is to honor all births as beautiful, important, and worth telling.

In this book, I offer a menu of supportive prompts, suggestions, and guidance in the hopes that you will discover what is most useful and inspiring to you. As you read this book, I recommend keeping a Birth Story Journal in which you can complete the Journal Activities offered throughout the book. While this book is designed to be read from start to finish, I know the reality of parenting time doesn't typically afford us hours of leisurely reading. Therefore, feel free to seek out what you are looking for at any given reading opportunity—perhaps you read a birth story (noted by the grey-to-the-edge pages), complete a writing prompt or several (in simple lined boxes throughout), or explore some aspect of birth story-writing that inspires you today. May this book be accessible and useful to you personally.

More than anything, my deep wish is that you benefit greatly from processing your story through writing. May you come to experience the value in your own storytelling, the power of your voice as you express your most profound life experiences and a deep honoring of your birth, no matter what it looked like.

I welcome you on this journey to remember, process, heal, and honor your birth.

Because your story matters.

PART ONE

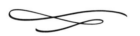

Why Write?

CHAPTER ONE

We are Storytellers

*There is no greater agony than
bearing an untold story inside you.*
MAYA ANGELOU

OR MOST OF HUMAN HISTORY, storytelling was the most potent way to transmit knowledge and wisdom among kin. We actually depended on it to survive, and in some regards, we still do. Until recently, the wisdom of childbirth has been a central narrative to our personal and communal lives. For most of time, women who'd reached childbearing age had witnessed the births of siblings, relatives, friends, and neighbors. They'd listened to birth stories around fires at dusk, heard the courageous cries of birthing women at sunrise, and woven the wisdom of birth into the fabric of their lives.

Birth was normal and natural. It wasn't removed from life—it was life. Somewhere along the way, we became severed from our deep connection to this collective wisdom.

We are still in the recovery process.

Many of our grandmothers (and perhaps even our mothers) were put under anesthesia, "twilight sleep," during labor—not to mention they were typically bed-bound, shaved, shot up, and sliced through by the time baby let out her first cry. Generations of women have been disconnected and disempowered in their experience of birth. If women even remembered their births, it wasn't likely they spoke about them with any sense of agency or accomplishment.

Still today, globally and in our own backyards, many women have few options or control over their birth experiences. It can almost feel taboo to speak candidly about birth, much less to own and honor our experience. While we may feel discouraged from sharing our stories, we also have a deep longing in our bones—set there by generations of story-sharing ancestors—to tell our truths. As one mother in the birth story anthology *Labor Day* reflects, "I entered this new world of motherhood tentatively, a little fawn-like teetering on unsure legs. [. . .] One thing I knew for sure: I wanted to talk about the birth. I wanted to tell what happened. I wanted this with a fervor that felt almost biological."[1]

I've repeatedly witnessed the deep longing women have to tell their stories of birth. Last summer I attended a writing retreat in France with a handful of women from around the world. After settling into my room at the sizable chateau, I travelled down the winding iron staircase and padded softly in my brown leather sandals along a simple dirt path to a communal table in the yard. Sitting, I was quickly offered a glass of rosé and a smattering of roasted vegetables to calm my growing traveler's hunger. This was my kind of place.

Blonde and kohl-eyed, wise and fascinating, Marilene, a radiant woman in her late sixties, turned toward me and introduced herself. She was from Indianapolis and had worked professionally as an intuitive therapist, healer, and spiritual teacher for more than four decades. She'd had her own TV shows and radio programs. But one detail she shared stood out: "I remember my birth."

My right eyebrow perked up as it does when I am intrigued, and I silently held space for this thread of her story to unravel further.

"I don't mean the story of my son's birth, of course I remember that. I mean I remember my own birth."

"Wow," was about the best I could muster. "Tell me more about that."

Marilene proceeded to tell the story of her own birth. "I can remember being so excited to be born," she recalls. "I remember the faces of everyone in that room. My mother was given ether in the hospital; that's what they did back then. As I got to her face, I thought she was dead. I mean, she really looked dead. It was so scary."

"Wow," I said again. "I'll bet that was incredibly scary. It's amazing that you have access to that memory." And I thought, as I have many times, about our children's experience entering this world. We may not all have conscious access to the memory of our own births, but it surely has profound power and influence in our unconscious, where many pre-verbal experiences are held.

As with group conversations, the story at the table shifted as more voices entered the fold. Not five minutes after Marilene shared her story, the darling chateau owner emerged from the kitchen and joined our conversation. Karolina, originally from Poland, is the kind of woman who can make a plain black tee shirt and humble A-line skirt look like runway attire. As her two small children played nearby, Karolina began telling her daughter's birth story as naturally as if she were introducing herself.

"She was so big when she was born," she said, referring to the little blonde angel who'd stopped affixing feathers to her toy car to sneak a mama-snuggle.

"I've never felt safe in a hospital, so I knew that wasn't the place for me to give birth. We were living in Turkey on a boat at the time and I planned to give birth on the boat. I had a doctor, midwife, and doula all come on the boat. I really wanted a natural birth, this was so important to me," she continued in her endearing accent.

"She was so big and she didn't want to come. I labored on the boat for a long time—for five hours, contractions came a minute apart and I was so exhausted." She paused and looked around the table.

"Did you know that the cesarean rate in Turkey is eighty percent? Women want to plan their births so they can manage what comes along after," she said, with sadness in her voice.

"So I went to the hospital. I felt down and touched my baby's head. She was so close, but she didn't want to come! I gave birth to her naturally after twenty-two hours of labor. She was four and a half kilograms—what is that? Ten pounds? She was a big baby," she laughed with both triumph and exhaustion in her voice. I could feel all the complex emotions held snugly between the story's spoken words.

Before our afternoon snack time had ended, another woman in our group, Leah, told the story of her own daughter, whom she'd adopted. Leah spoke of her and her husband's desire to have a child; of the long, discouraging adoption process they'd endured in seeking a child from outside the US; the insight her friend Marilene had given her about looking for a child domestically; and the wildly unexpected call from a pregnant woman who'd found Leah's adoption profile online and wanted to explore the possibility of adoption with her.

"I couldn't believe we had made a connection and we might actually be bringing our child home in less than a month. It was so surreal and so amazing."

Later, under the blazing Bordeaux sun, I dipped my toes into the sparkling azure waters of the chateau's backyard swimming pool and thought about the birth stories I'd heard in the short time we women had been together. Given my work around birth I wondered if I was simply a magnet for birth stories. But then I thought of all the different times and situations where I'd witnessed a similar kind of birth story sharing. And it was suddenly so clear to me: when women gather, we tell stories. And we have this insatiable natural desire to express and remember our experiences of birth, these incredibly powerful stories that have shaped our lives. We can't *not* share these stories.

We must tell our stories. Because they are important. Because we are important.

Because our children are important. The love we feel for our children is incomparable to any other love we feel in this lifetime—and birth is the opening chapter of that epic love story.

A birth story is the personal equivalent of the creation story that every civilization throughout time has constructed to make meaning of its collective experience. Consider the birth of Gaia in Greek mythology, Mary's birth of Jesus, and all the origin stories of cultures throughout time and space. We have a deep longing to know how we came to be and a deep need to share the incredible stories of bringing a child into this world.

A birth story is also a heroine's story—it is often the story of a woman overcoming her fears and great obstacles to emerge on the other side alive and with new gifts. It is also a journey that brings great challenge and risk.

As Jalaja Bonheim writes, "Giving birth is priestess work; it requires a woman to pass through a painful and dangerous initiation in which she journeys to the threshold between worlds and risks her own life to help another soul cross over."[2]

A birth story is a profound rite of passage—we are forever changed by our transformation from maiden to mother. Birth is the first thread in the tapestry of our lives, and when a new birth is added to our tapestry it changes the texture of everything that came before and everything that will come after.

Our stories are so important, yet how often is the mothering voice silenced and marginalized in our culture? We do the most miraculous work of humanity in soft whispers behind closed doors. This quiet, humble side of mothering—the best kept secret of humanity—is beautiful in its hushed tones, yet our stories must be sung—they are such a valuable aspect of our personal and collective human experience. They deserve to be seen and shared. They *need* to be seen and shared.

Author, doula, and childbirth educator Penny Simkin, in her study about the long-term influence of birth on a woman's life, concludes: "It is clear that the birth experience has a powerful effect on women[,] with a potential for permanent or long-term positive or negative impact."[3]

Our births indeed have a powerful effect on many aspects of our lives, including how we feel about ourselves, our bodies, our identity, our relationships—with our child, our partner, our family, and other mothers—and life itself. Author Arielle Greenberg writes, "My first two births made me. They are the experiences that have most deeply shaped every choice I've made, every path I've taken since."[4]

Birth is also a profound rite of passage and hero's journey for fathers and partners, which we explore further in Chapter 7.

CHAPTER TWO

We Write to Remember

We write to taste life twice, in the moment and in retrospect.
ANAÏS NIN

—————

A T ITS SIMPLEST, writing down your birth story helps you remember and record what it was like to give birth (or witness your partner give birth)—capturing and preserving these life-altering moments.

In the days following birth, you may run through your birth story again and again in your mind, remembering all the little details. This is when you recall so easily the feel of the blanket under which you labored at home, the taste of the pepperoni pizza you inhaled two hours after baby was born, the look on your partner's face when s/he first set eyes on baby, the words people spoke during birth, what was happening inside as you reached transition, the song you heard between contractions, the kind of car you drove to the hospital, the name of your favorite nurse, the day of the week and the weather, the gaze of your newborn child the first time you nursed. But as time goes on, many of these details inevitably fade from our memories. It is the nature of the human brain. We don't think it will happen, but slowly these details vanish from our conscious minds and we are left with a fragment of the original.

While accessing the minutia of your birth experience may be easiest in those early days, it is never too late. When we begin to we write, we begin to remember; even if your birth feels out of reach because you don't remember it clearly, writing will help you access what you'd thought you'd lost.

What's amazing about memory is that once you set the intention to explore a past experience, it can be like opening a book you'd read long ago—you could only recall vague details until you turned that first page, and then suddenly you could recollect all manner of specifics as they became illuminated on the pages of your mind.

Not only can writing help us remember by offering an external record of the event, the act of writing enhances our internal memory of the event. Writing utilizes our brains and memories in a different way than speaking. The act of writing stimulates a collection of cells in the brainstem called the Reticular Activating System (RAS), which acts like the brain's nightclub bouncer, checking the IDs of all incoming information to decide what gets in and what is worthy of our conscious attention. Writing something down sends a message to the brain that this content is important—VIP if you will—and worthy of special care.

We remember what we write down better than what we simply think or say to another person.

Writing can also serve to mark a point in time, to preserve the memory of our perspective at any given moment. (We further explore how time alters our stories on page 147.)

This can be especially helpful as we use writing in the process of exploring our birth experience. Kelsey, who shares her story on page 141, reflects on the power of capturing our memories of birth as they change through time:

> *Were I to write my story at different points in time, the events I would highlight and the meanings I would make would inevitably vary. I find that fascinating and useful— what was the story when I was in initial shock and awe?*

How did I story it when the doubt and self-judgment set in? When I was grappling with the trauma of certain parts? After I had worked through all that? The story is dynamic and alive and the ways it is told at different points can be hugely informative over time.

Thus, we can use writing to remember not just what happened at our birth, but how we felt about it and what it meant to us, then and onward, as we journey through the process of exploring and integrating our experience.

CHAPTER THREE

We Write to Process

I don't know what I think until I write about it.
JOAN DIDION

———————

THIS ACT OF WRITING to *remember* our birth experience points to the power in using writing to *process and reflect*. Most women (and many men, I suspect!) have a strong desire to process their birth stories in one way or another. But not all have the permission (self-given or otherwise), time, space, or tools to fully process their experience. Life moves swiftly forward following birth. If we don't take time to process our experience, it can remain undigested or partially digested, which can compromise our overall vitality in ways we may not even be aware of. Writing gives us the time, space, and tools to process what happened and digest our experiences in a way not possible through other forms of expression.

So how exactly do we process our birth experiences through writing? In processing our birth stories, we review and reflect on the events surrounding our birth—what happened, where, how, and when—exploring how we felt in those moments and now, and drawing meaning from our births, our bodies, ourselves, others, and life itself. It's an exploration of all three layers of a birth story, which are described in detail in Chapter Ten.

Why is processing our birth experience important? Why do we do it? By processing our stories through writing, we gain a sense of order, clarity, and understanding about our experiences. We can also find a safe place in writing to explore, discover, sort, and find support for our thoughts and feelings about our births. Processing our births through writing allows us to shift our perspectives, make meaning and integrate our birth experiences into the fabric of who we are. As one mother notes, "Writing is how I sort out my emotions, make meaning of the events that happened, and sift the experience for new understandings it has to offer. Otherwise, the thoughts and emotions just swirl around my head in a jumbled mess."

Writing offers us the perfect context in which to gain a sense of order, clarity, and understanding about our births.

The narrative structure's inherent design invites such processing. Through writing, we begin to get a sense of the chronology of our experience, making order from what may have seemed intense and jumbled at the outset. We also gain clarity as we write. *Did this happen? How did it happen? Oh, then this happened, that makes sense.* And so on.

Writing helps us slow our story down long enough to gain understanding about what happened. While spoken words come and go like the breeze, writing suspends our thoughts in mid-air—so that we may turn them over, inspect them from different angles, and discover a subtle code lying faintly between the lines. Writing gives our words lifespan—it allows them to live outside of us long enough for us to see and discover something in them.

This slowing down required by writing cultivates an exploration and discovery of our inner landscape—our thoughts, emotions, and needs. Exploring the narrative structure of our stories gives us an opportunity to work through some of the deeper threads hidden beneath the veneer of our labor chronology.

For many women, so much is at stake through the pregnancy and birth process. Pressures to perform a certain way or live up to birthing ideals (set by ourselves or others), thoughts and beliefs about our bodies; our ability to love ourselves and others; our interdependence and autonomy; our sense of agency over our own lives; our values, courage, voice, vulnerability, surrender, faith, truth—all of these are possible themes we have the opportunity to explore and work through as we process our birth experiences through writing. (See Appendix A for a list of possible birth story themes.)

We also have the opportunity to make discoveries and connections that may not otherwise reveal themselves. Sometimes we think that writing is just about *documenting* our experiences, but what we find is that we *discover* something rich and valuable we never knew before. Kelsey writes:

> *I didn't initially see how each of my births was connected. It sounds kind of unfathomable, but prior to writing about my third birth, I hadn't fully realized how much my first birth (D&C) had affected my second (live) birth. I hadn't realized how much incredible courage it took to even give birth again, and to birth with as much tenacity as I did. For years after the second birth, I shamed and blamed myself for not being brave enough to dilate and strong enough to birth without meds.*

> *As I connected those two births in writing, I stepped back, suddenly seeing, "Oh, mama. Oh, sweet mama! Of course you were terrified! Of course you held onto that baby as though both of your lives depended on it! You birthed with as much courage, bravery, strength, and tenacity as any other woman! Who cares what the outcome was; you birthed from within, with all you had. You were and are a birth*

warrior." I felt this huge surge of compassion and tenderness
for myself, and all the judgment and shame faded away.

We see how writing enabled Kelsey to gain greater clarity and connection about her births, cultivate self-empathy, and heal heavier emotions like shame and harsh internal criticism.

For those of us who may struggle in processing our birth experiences, writing can remove the burden of carrying our stories in silence.

The written word is stable, sturdy, and strong.
It can handle the weight of your world.

When you write about something heavy or hard, it's as if the words are bearing witness to your woes and slowly siphoning the sadness from your heart. Writing allows you to become a witness to your own tender experiences. As a witness, you have the opportunity to see yourself in all your humanity and to offer love, compassion, understanding, and acceptance. (See Appendix F on page 277 for a tool that can further help you cultivate self-empathy through writing.)

Billy, whose story appears on page 47, reflects on the discoveries, connections, and healing he experienced by processing his story: "Through writing, I shined a light on my own shame around the birth of my son. And shame cannot exist in the light." Writing about his son's birth yielded unique benefits he hadn't experienced in nearly two decades of talking about his experience.

As these writers' reflections reveal, we not only discover something new through writing, but we can dramatically change our relationship to our past and to ourselves. Through writing, we can revisit, review, and even rewrite our past. What we thought happened—what we believe happened to us—can shift and change as we reveal deeper and more complex truths. It's not that we use writing to deny our experiences, but we use writing to shift our perspective. Writing has the power to help us discover and choose what meaning and power our stories hold.

Betsy, whose story appears below, was also surprised at the discoveries she made in writing her son's birth story nearly three decades after his birth. In fact, in writing about his birth, she healed a piece of her own birth.

BETSY'S STORY

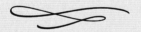

"The doctor said my water broke."

The other end of the line was silent.

"Butch, you there?"

"Yes." It was my husband's voice, but it was much quieter than I was used to.

"Is he sure?" Butch asked, barely audible.

"Of course, he's sure!v I said. "He said to call you and let you know they are admitting me to the birthing center. Do you remember where it is?"

The other end of the line was quiet again.

"I don't think I can drive," he said. "I think I'm going to be sick."

This was not the response I was expecting from the soon-to-be father of my first baby. Butch had avoided all the birthing classes. "Too busy," he said, so I went by myself. I left a copy of *What to Expect When You're Expecting* around the house, hoping he would try and inform himself. I didn't mind his absence at the classes. I could take care of myself.

"Hold on," I said. I was making the call from the nurses' station at my doctor's office. This was 1990, before we had cell phones. I had come in for a check-up after waking up that morning with liquid running down my leg. My husband, Butch, had left three hours earlier to be on-air for his morning radio show. I thought the liquid might be pee, but I called my godfather Bill, a doctor, to get his advice.

"It was only a small amount of liquid, and there hasn't been anymore," I told him. "I feel fine. No contractions." I was only thirty-eight weeks, our house was being renovated, and I had lunch plans with some friends. I was not ready to have a baby. Not today.

"You should still call your doctor's office. You're almost thirty-eight weeks and it could be amniotic fluid," he replied. "You don't want to take any chances. Call us and let us know what the doctor says." My godmother, Betty, was on the other line at the house with Bill. "I love you Betty Jane," she said to me before they hung up. She was the only person who called me that; I was named after her, but my name was changed to Betsy. "I love you too, Betty Jane."

Back at the doctor's office, I stood at the nurses' station and held my hand over the receiver as I spoke to the nurse. "My husband doesn't think he can drive. When I told him it was time to have the baby, he said he felt sick. Do you mind if I take my car to go pick him up?"

The nurse shook her head. "You really shouldn't be driving. Let me check with the doctor."

I don't know why I didn't think to call Butch a taxi or have someone else bring him, or why it suddenly became my problem to get him to the birthing center when I was the one having the baby. I also wanted to go home and get a few things. I didn't leave the house that day expecting to be a mother when I returned.

The nurse reappeared. "The doctor said you can go pick up your husband as long as you drive straight back."

"Thanks, I'll be back in forty-five minutes."

"Don't come back to the office," the nurse added. "Go straight to the birthing center. They're holding a bed for you."

I got into my white Volvo sedan and drove across town to our home. The house was in the midst of a renovation and was supposed to be done in another two weeks.

My expected due date was January 24, 1990. That day was January 3. I didn't have a kitchen or a room for the baby ready. My nieces,

Daisy and Poppy, were visiting from England over their school holiday. They were thrilled when they heard I was going to have the baby early.

"What do you think you're having?" Daisy asked.

"I don't know," I said. "What do you think?"

Nine years old, Poppy leaned forward and spoke to my stomach. "I can't wait to meet you, baby Griswold," she whispered.

I let our dogs, Elvis and Dean, out while I waited for Butch. Someone from work was going to drop him at the house. I moved slowly as I packed a bag for the hospital. I still didn't feel like I was in labor but suddenly I moved like I was.

Butch walked through the back door looking like he was going to pass out.

"What do we do now?" he said anxiously.

"I've already packed," I said, "and Laura is coming to watch the girls. We just need to get back to the hospital."

"I'll call Mark and see how soon he can get the house done," Butch said, like that was the priority.

"Should I boil water or something for the car ride?" he asked. "Or warm towels?"

"The doctor said I'm in the early stages; my cervix is barely dilated."

"I have no idea what that means," he said.

"You would if you'd come to the baby classes," I smiled.

"Blood and body fluids make me sick," he said.

"Let's go have a baby," I said as I opened the passenger door for him.

We checked into the hospital and then waited and waited. I had only leaked a small amount of amniotic fluid earlier in the day. The nurse said that as soon as the rest of the fluid was released, my labor would be quicker. For now, I was comfortable, with no strong contractions.

"Maybe you should start the special breathing," Butch said, forcefully inhaling and exhaling though his mouth.

"That's not until the baby is ready to come. Did you watch that on some show?"

"Maybe," he smiled. "I know a few things."

"I'm going to check on the girls," he added, and he quickly left the room. Butch could never sit still very long. He always had to be on the move, running errands.

After twelve hours in the hospital, I was hungry and tired. The nurse brought me more ice chips.

"I think you're going to be here for the night," the doctor said as he checked me one last time before he went home.

A few hours earlier, a nurse had manually broken my water to speed up the labor. She reached inside me and poked a hole in the amniotic sac. It was odd the way hands were going in and out of me without asking permission, the staff just telling me what they were going to do. I had wanted a doula or midwife but that was considered too hippie at the time, at least to Butch. "Let's let the professionals handle this," was his response.

My cervix was still barely dilated, but the contractions began to get stronger. I wanted a natural birth but my body was exhausted. The doctor suggested I get an epidural to ease the pain. I agreed. My excitement for giving birth turned to exhaustion.

I sat up on the side of the bed as the anesthesiologist stuck a needle through my spine. It tingled and then sent a wave of nausea through me. I leaned forward and Butch offered me a tray to catch the vomit. He looked away from the tray and me. His eyes were wide as he looked at the epidural shot. "That's a big prick," he said to the doctor and then they started joking with each other. I glared at both of them until they stopped. This was not his comedy show.

I lay on my side and tried to sleep during the night, interrupted every hour or so by a nurse who came to check me.

"Still no baby?" the doctor said when he checked on me the next morning. It had been almost twenty-four hours. "You're beginning to dilate more, so I promise you'll have a baby sometime today. The epidural will keep you comfortable."

The drugs flowing through my body were so powerful, I couldn't feel my feet. Every twenty minutes or so, a band of energy across my back and belly tightened but otherwise I didn't feel much.

Butch had left me sometime during the early morning hours. He seemed fine to drive so he drove my car to the radio station to host his four-hour morning show. He needed to stay busy. I needed calm. He passed by the hospital at the end of his show. He entered the room as the nurse had her gloved hand inside my vagina, checking my cervix.

"How dilated is she?" he said to the nurse. After nearly thirty hours of labor, he was suddenly an expert on the lingo. "And where do I scrub?" he added, holding his hands up.

"You can wash your hands in the sink," the nurse smiled. "And she's at seven centimeters but her contractions are still far apart, so it won't be anytime soon but it will be today."

Butch washed his hands and then walked towards the front of the bed, careful not to glance at the nurse as she removed her hand. Since I arrived to give birth, he had managed to avoid looking at my genitals.

Our doctor sauntered in. He spoke like he was a cowboy just off his horse. "Let me check you," he said as he put a glove on his right hand and pushed his hand inside me all in one motion. His eyes looked towards the ceiling as he reached for my cervix. I felt nothing, just some pressure.

"You're still at seven," he said. "I'm getting concerned about the baby. It's been almost thirty hours—that can be hard on the baby. I think it's best if we do a cesarean section."

My heart sank. I'd avoided even reading about C-sections. They were never an option. I wanted to have a natural birth. At this point, it wasn't even natural because of this heavy epidural. Were my feet supposed to be numb too?

"Right now?" Butch said. "The baby is coming now?"

"No, we'll need some time to prep her," the doc said.

"Okay, I need to go get my nieces. I promised them I'd take them to a movie," Butch replied. "I'll drop them at the movies and be back in an hour."

Butch, off for an errand, again.

The room got quiet after everyone left. I took a few moments to hold my baby from the outside. I didn't know what I'd be having. It would be a surprise. I sent the baby a message and said I'm ready for you to come into the world. I sent my body a message and said I want to give birth naturally. Monitors were around my stomach, recording my vitals. I could watch the baby's heartbeat across a screen.

I'd listened to the heartbeat in the doctor's office for the first time when the baby was about sixteen weeks old. I told Butch about it when I got home. The sound reminded me of the first time I heard my own heartbeat. I was five, and my godfather was listening to my heartbeat as he checked me when I was sick. Growing up, I rarely went to a doctor's office. When I was sick, I would call my godparents and they would tend to me until I was better.

When I asked what my heart sounded like, Bill put the earbuds of his stethoscope to my ears. *Swoosh, swoosh, swoosh*, I heard. Then he moved the scope to his heart. I called my godmother so I could hear her heart. We all sounded the same.

My mom gave birth to me just before lunch on February 5, 1963.

The day after my birth, it was discovered that my three older siblings had chicken pox so my godparents, Betty and Bill, offered to take me to their house and care for me until my siblings were better. My parents didn't protest, especially since their home shared a backyard divided by a fence with my godparent's home. I'd be nearby. Two days later, my mom went home with my dad, and I went home with Betty and Bill. Their teenage daughters, Wendy and Cathy, were waiting on the front porch to meet me. I can imagine myself smiling up at the four of them gazing at me reverently while I'm thinking, "Now this is more like it."

After two weeks, my mom tried to take me home, but Betty, a nurse, and Bill, a doctor, who had both served during the war, inspected the nearly healed chicken pox on my siblings and told Mom, "We'd better keep Betsy a few more weeks just to be safe,v like it was a war zone at the Blankenbaker house.

Later I found out that Betty's third child, a girl named Judy, was delivered stillborn at full term. Betty was put to sleep for the delivery and when she woke up and found out her baby was dead, she didn't want to see her. Eight years after she refused to hold her dead baby, I was placed in Betty's arms. "After you were born and named after Mom, she felt like she got another chance to be a mother," Cathy told me. "You were the reason my parents were able to move forward after losing Judy."

Betty and Bill usually spent winters in Florida to avoid the cold in Indiana. When they found out I was going to give birth, they packed up and began the sixteen-hour drive to Indianapolis. I was still in labor when they arrived.

As I was being prepped for C-section, I told the nurse I felt a pressure; I felt like pushing. She looked at my cervix, and I watched her eyes get big. "Hold on, let me call the doctor. Don't push."

The doctor walked in the room a minute later, pulling on his green scrubs. "Looks like you're going to get your wish. The baby is ready to come out."

Butch isn't here, I thought.

"Pull your legs back, and when I tell you, push," said the nurse. I grabbed behind my thighs and felt a band of pressure around my abdomen.

"Okay, Betsy, time to push," the doctor said.

I took a deep breath and. . .

Butch walked in the room. He couldn't help but take a look at my wide-open genitals. "Is this a C-section?" he said as he put his hands in the air. "Where do I scrub?"

"No, she's having the baby naturally," the nurse said as she left me and walked over to put a gown and gloves on Butch.

"Good work, Betsy," the doctor said. "You can stop pushing. You're almost there."

I looked over at Butch and he had gone pale. Another nurse left me and helped ease him into a rocking chair that I suppose is for when the baby is born. "Let's have you sit down for a moment."

"What do I do next?" he asked as his knees began to buckle.

"Why don't you sit for a minute? Let me get you some juice," the nurse said.

"You're going to be a father here real soon," the doctor added.

I looked at the now trio as they tended to my husband. "I feel like I'm ready to push again," I said.

"Okay, Betsy," said the doctor. "Here you go. Steady breaths as you push. Good girl. A little more. The baby's head is coming out. Lots of hair. Keep pushing."

I looked at Butch in the rocking chair. The color had come back to his cheeks. He stood up and walked to the end of the bed, eyes fully on my pelvic area.

"Good work, Betsy. Almost there," whispered the nurses.

Butch and I both took an inhale at the same time and with the exhale, I pushed until the baby emerged and my body went from carrying two heartbeats, mine and the baby's, to only one.

Butch reached down to help catch the baby.

"It's a boy," he said.

I smiled and reached for the baby, but he was taken away to be tested, cleaned, and bundled. Then he was handed to Butch, who carried him to the rocking chair and sat staring at him and talking to him.

"Welcome to the world, little buddy. I'm your daddy," he rocked slowly. "And that's your mommy. And we're your family, the Griswolds."

Reflecting on her writing, Betsy is awed by the healing that came through about her own birth and her experience with her godmother Betty. "Through writing, I suddenly made the connection: my presence in Betty's home as a newborn was healing for her. It allowed her to offer that love she wanted to give to her own child to me. It really shifted a lot for me around my own birth."

And it wasn't just her own birth that she received healing from. "After writing down the story of my first child's birth, I sent him (Sam) a long email—not just about his birth, but about his life, our family, my divorce from his father, all of it. We connected in a way we hadn't before, and it healed some of my past regrets around my divorce."

Exploring what we think and how we feel about our births is important because they weave together to form the stories of our lives.

Our very identity is the accumulation of stories we tell ourselves about who we are.

Writing gives us a space to tell our stories with intentionality, reflection, and purpose—enabling us to have agency over who we are. How we choose to process and remember our stories determines whether the transformational power of birth serves or hinders our own personal growth.

CHAPTER FOUR

We Write to Claim

And when I need to work anything out, I turn to the blank page.
There, no one can steal my pain or try to claim my knowing.
And there, I always have the final word in my own story.
GLENNON DOYLE

———————

BIRTH REQUIRES SOME OF THE GREATEST SURRENDER we'll ever experience. So much of the birth process is ultimately out of our control. We may set our intentions and make our preferences known, but what happens does not always follow our carefully dreamt plans. In some cases, others have made choices during our births that have profoundly shaped our stories—and they don't feel like our own. In many cases, birth is so intense and powerful that we feel as if it were something that happened *to* us, rather than something in which we had an active role.

Regardless of the degree to which we feel we own our experience, writing our stories down is a way to claim or reclaim our births as our own.

You may not have been able to control some aspects of your birth, but you are in complete control over the story. You get to decide what gets written.

You get to decide what details are highlighted, what is less important to you. You get to interpret the experience and decide what it means. You get to write exactly how you feel, and how you felt.

You get to say, "This is mine."

Not only can writing offer us a way to claim our *experience*, it also allows us to become fully sovereign over our *story*. Writing down your story offers you a *space of your own* that doesn't need to be shared with anyone. Writing does not require a social context and is unaffected by listeners. You don't have to edit or filter depending on an audience, which we all do to some degree when we speak with another person.

When we write our stories, no one is there to comment, criticize, or curtail the way we tell our stories. This makes writing a safe and free place for us to be as we truly are. Our defenses can come down. We can say what we truly want to say. Our stories can be ours.

One mother of three reflects on the difference between telling and writing her story:

> I've found that most people aren't that interested in hearing about the soul work of birth. Most listeners want the quick facts—hours of labor, method of delivery, the comical parts, baby's stats—and keep it under five minutes! It's a rare bird or bestie that wants to know what your soul went through—your moments of greatest darkness, your moments of greatest triumph, the song playing as they started your Pitocin drip, what your partner said when you were begging for it to stop.
>
> Most people want to know what they want to know, not what you want to tell them. This is why is it's extra important to write about birth—so you get to tell it the way you

want to tell it, whether that's a recounting of every gritty detail or some sweeping symbolic poetry.

For this mother, and many other parents, writing is a way to tell the soul of their story in a way not possible through other means.

For those who have experienced a difficult birth, telling the story to others can prove difficult or stifling. Consider Mary Beth Keane's reflection on how it feels to share her story with other women:

> *Even now, four years later, when I exchange birth stories with other women, often someone says, "But you had an epidural!" and I see that person dismiss my story entirely. Or they say, "But you didn't have a transfusion. You couldn't have lost that much blood." Or they counter my story with a story about someone who had an emergency hysterectomy. Or worse. Sometimes I see in other women an impatience with my story of a difficult birth, and they go in the opposite direction and describe how easy it was for them.* [5]

Through writing, we are free from the comparisons, the discounting, the evaluations.

We can just tell our stories. If telling your story feels vulnerable, raw, confusing, or difficult, you can trust a piece of paper. When you hate what you wrote, you can take it back or change it, unlike with spoken words.

You can write your story and burn it and no one ever has to know about it. You can also write your story and shout it from the mountaintops.

You get to decide.

AUBREY'S STORY

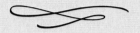

My journey of birthing children began in the United States. I had my two older boys, Owen and Ethan, in a hospital. Their births went well: I had the standard obstetrician and standard medical care, I went along with whatever the doctor told me, and that was that. I had both of them naturally, drug-free. We moved to Australia in January 2006 and a couple of years later I became a doula, which opened my eyes to amazing possibilities. My husband and I decided we were ready for a third and it was a very exciting time for our family. We immediately decided to take charge of this birth and have a home birth. My pregnancy was beautiful; my children and husband were involved every step of the way.

On June 25, my husband Torin and I were watching television together, and at about 9:00 p.m. I felt a little gush of water. I was shocked because my previous labors had not started this way. I went to the bathroom to make sure, and I was pretty confident this was it! It was six days before my estimated due date. I called my doula, Susan, straight away and she said to take it easy, rest, drink, and see what happens. An hour and a half later my surges started, and I was leaking more fluid. I called my midwife, Jane, to let her know and that I would keep her posted. My labors usually lasted only about four to five hours, so she knew to be ready. Torin was very calm and let me do whatever I needed. I was so excited.

I stayed in the kitchen for the most part, stopping between surges and leaning on a chair, rocking back and forth. Torin kept the heat packs coming. Jane arrived about midnight and was a wonderful, peaceful presence in our home. Soon after, Susan and our student midwife Melanie arrived. Everyone surrounded me with peace and support. Torin filled the pool, and that brought great relief. Susan was a rock star when it came to making sure I had a cold cloth on my head at all times.

When I was in the pool, everything went calm: Torin kept rubbing my head, Susan and Jane drifted in and out of light sleep, Melanie was knitting. It was very comforting that everyone was so calm. I was still getting surges but it was such a gift to have this rest before the real work began!

After probably a good thirty to forty-five minutes of this very quiet time, I was quickly reminded of being in labor. My urge to push was very strong and very real. In my previous labors at the hospital, they were constantly checking my dilation, and once I was ten centimeters dilated, they told me to push; I never once had the urge. Well I can now say I know what it is like. It took over my entire body. We knew we would meet our little one very soon, so I asked Torin to go and get the boys up. They had been sleeping up until that point. They eagerly woke up and knew right away what was going on. Our birth pool was positioned between two lounges, and they both curled up together with great anticipation. I was making quite a bit of laboring noise, which startled my oldest, Owen. The wonderful thing was after each surge and push, I would stop and talk with my children, letting them know I was okay and the sounds I was making were helping the baby come.

They were the first to see the head appear and we were all so excited, and then came our beautiful baby. Torin reached down and caught him and handed him right to me. I felt immediately that it was a boy, and I announced right away. We were all shocked because we had been convinced it was a girl, but I was instantly overjoyed that I had my three boys.

Tasman Raymond Torin Wicks was born at 3:30 a.m.; he weighed seven and a half pounds.

I held our new little baby for quite some time and just enjoyed the moment we had all just shared. Owen held his brother for about an hour while I birthed the placenta and got cleaned up. Tasman took my breast naturally, at his own pace, with no nurses forcing him on or monitoring our every move. What a blessed experience.

I was soon tucked into bed with my bundle. It was about 6:00 a.m. and we all had a long sleep.

In closing my birth story of Tasman, I have to say this birth experience was unbelievable and all that I could ever imagine. All of my births were, of course, but this one was something really special, in our home surrounded by love and my children; there is nothing like it. My midwives, Jane and Melanie, were fantastic— they gave me just the space and respect that I needed. My doula, Susan, empowered me in so many ways, in training me as a doula and being there reminding me along the way that I was doing well.

As Aubrey writes in the opening of this story, she "went along with whatever the doctor told [her], and that was that" with her first two births. With her third birth, she really stakes a claim to her birth experiences and becomes more of an agent and director of her care, advocating for and receiving the support she needs on her terms. And we see how important that was for her (as it is for all of us: to receive the support we need, on our terms). Writing about her birth was another way to express that sovereignty over her body and her birth.

Sometimes we stake our claim to our stories in a celebratory spirit and other times that claiming or reclaiming process is a whole lot grittier and hard-earned. Even when birth doesn't go well and we write about it, we can begin to claim sovereignty over our story, to claim the telling of it and the making of its meaning.

CHAPTER FIVE

We Write to Heal

I would say my first two births carried trauma, and writing about them helped heal my wounds and bring me back to awareness of my own capabilities.

KELSEY STARRS

WRITING ABOUT BIRTH OFFERS us all an opportunity for healing, even those of us who don't consider our births traumatic. All births carry some degree of intensity, and the birth journey requires such tremendous change and surrender. Writing provides a safe and effective container for us to explore and express emotions like shock, grief, ambivalence, anger, and sorrow—that may be difficult to otherwise express—so that we can integrate them into the fabric of our being and so that they don't linger undigested to show up in a new form down the road.

While writing can help all of us process and heal intense aspects of our births, writing is particularly valuable for processing more significant traumas associated with them. Birth trauma can have different origins and take on different forms for each of us, as we've already seen in Kelsey's and Billy's comments about writing their birth stories in Chapter Three. Our births themselves can be traumatic, we may experience trauma as a result of birth loss, past traumas can surface during our births, and we may experience trauma stemming from what surrounds our births, such as difficult relationships and other aspects of our lives.

We look at each of these kinds of birth trauma below in greater detail, but let's first explore the benefits of writing as a way to heal. When we experience something as traumatic, the innate intelligence of our being seeks ways to process and digest this experience. This may manifest as recurrent dreams, intrusive thoughts, intense emotions, an intense desire to share (or, conversely, to suppress), physical symptoms signaling discord in our beings, and more. While it may seem like adding insult to injury, these are attempts to create opportunities for personal healing.

Most of us experience these as uncomfortable and even overwhelming, so instead of trusting and leaning into these innate impulses, we pull away, stuff down, numb, avoid, and reject. We often lack permission or a safe container to explore our traumas. Still, the body and soul yearn for the expression of what is *true*, however painful.

Repressing our traumas takes a major toll on our well-being. On the physical level this repression can compromise our immune systems, reduce our capacity to fight off infections, increase our risk of heart problems, interfere with sleep and digestion, cause headaches and body aches, alter hormones, decrease libido, and so much more. On the mental and emotional levels, repressing our traumas can cause irritability, anxiety, depression, and numbness. On a broader level, we can feel stuck and unable to move forward in our lives. We may be less able to show up fully in our lives in a way that feels good.

> The energy it takes to resist the truth is greater than the energy it takes to look it squarely in the eye and find safe ways to process, express, and move through it.

Over the last few years, I have been journeying through what I've experienced as trauma. Following my birth, I developed reproductive health problems that diminished my quality of life and threatened my ability to have more children. I spent a lot of energy resisting what was true, suppressing my grief and fear, and desperately trying to find a way out of the discomfort. As I traversed my own healing process, I began to recognize that the only way through this ordeal was *in* and *through* it. I couldn't go around it, I couldn't stay on the surface of it, I couldn't just stay where I was. I had to go all the way into the heart of this trauma and move through it.

At the time, the image of Mother Mary's Sacred Heart started showing up everywhere—it was referenced in books, magazines, and interviews; it showed up on walls, tee shirts, candles, paintings, restaurant menus, and even socks. That famous heart was everywhere. I do not consider myself particularly religious; in fact, I've had my own resistance around organized religion and its icons. But there she was, with her heart aflame, practically everywhere I looked. So I started to turn toward this recurring image and get curious. *Okay, Life, I'm paying attention, what is up with this heart on fire?*

Let's consider the heart: one of the first organs to develop in utero, it transmits the most powerful electromagnetic field in the body. Sixty-five percent of the heart is neurons, and it beats up to 40,000 times a day. What power, what intelligence, what devotion! In Sanskrit, the word for heart, *anahata*, means "unstuck" and is considered the place within us that is untouched by any wounding or trauma we experience in this lifetime. We also associate the heart with our emotions, and, for some, our souls.

Let's consider the fire. Fire is the element of transformation, purification, discipline, movement, passion, compassion, catharsis. It can keep us warm and facilitate nourishment, or it can destroy us. Fire can be the force that symbolically burns away all that is not true or that no longer serves us (as with the yogic concept of *tapas*).

The Sacred Heart was really the perfect symbol for me at the time. My health problems centered around my uterus, literally the "mother" organ, considered by some to be the body's "lower" heart. This heart became a symbol of my creative capacity; healing my relationship to "mother;" the presence and support of the Divine Mother; my expanding capacity to live from the heart and be willing to feel it all; a reminder of the initiatory, transformative power of fire and the birth/death/rebirth cycle; my own sacredness and the sacredness of my body; and the call to move all the way in and through my life experiences. The Sacred Heart's constant presence began to feel like a gift. It was a source of solace in an uncertain time and it remains a potent reminder of this journey and these lessons as a tattoo on my low belly, where my uterus once dwelled.

Among the rich symbolism of the Sacred Heart is a sword (or many) piercing through it. When I first began to connect to this image and to its symbolism for my own healing journey, I wanted to omit the sword. *Just more violence and destruction*, I thought. *No, thank you.* But then I began to understand what that sword meant. The sword is about piercing all the way into and through our emotions, our wounds, our suffering. It reminds us that we can't get to the place that is unstuck, that is untouched, that is whole, holy, and healed, by going away from or around our truths. We must go *in* and *through*.

Writing is a sword in the Sacred Mother's heart.

Writing offers a way into and through our wounding and our traumas as a means to heal.

Writing offers us a chance to symbolically represent our initial trauma with words, and in so doing, begin to honor that innate impulse to heal and move through our pain. We draw on the wisdom and benefits of our creativity and our imagination to support our more fundamental needs for safety, security, belonging, and well-being.

Writing will not eliminate our pain, but it can alter its effect on our lives. As Judith Harris writes, "Writing about painful experiences defends against the world-dissolving powers that often accompany trauma, depression, and mourning. When writing is healing, it can intercede for us by demonstrating our strength to confront our own pain without descending directly into the abyss or retreating into lethargy."[6] The memory of the pain is still there, but it doesn't rule or cripple our lives as it once did.

We can begin to see our own strengths, our own resiliency; we can begin to connect to self-compassion, empathy, and understanding. It can change everything.

The benefits of writing to heal are many, and as I see them, inextricably linked to the freedom from having to repress our truths. On the physical level, studies have shown that writing about trauma boosts the immune system and increases the body's capacity to fight off infection; it reduces the heart rate and brings the body into a more relaxed physiological state similar to those reached in yoga and meditation. It can produce behavioral changes and reduce anxiety and depression. Studies have found that writing can produce as much therapeutic benefit as therapy.

These benefits hold true whether or not you ever show your writing to someone else, and regardless of your perceived "skill" as a writer.

While the research overwhelmingly supports the profound benefits that can come with writing about trauma, there are a few caveats. It's not just any kind of writing that produces therapeutic benefits, but rather a certain approach or framework that is most useful (see Chapter 16, "Writing about Trauma").

It's also important to acknowledge that just because writing can help us heal doesn't mean it will be easy or comfortable. Touching on our deepest emotions and wounds can initially be difficult and uncomfortable, yet it can ultimately yield a greater outlook. Declaring "This happened to me and this is how I am feeling about it" is a powerful exercise on the healing path: this vulnerability and courage pave the way for ownership, connection, and empowerment. When we process the harder parts of our stories in writing, it can bring us into a greater awareness of ourselves, others, and the world that we couldn't have attained otherwise, helping us gain a more authentic perspective than ever before.

Lastly, and most importantly, writing about trauma is not a substitute for seeking professional support. I highly recommend using writing as an adjunct to the care of a highly trained professional support giver. This gives you a safe container to write and a place to seek support and guidance through the wildness of your wounding and out the other side.

Birth Trauma

Writing is a matter of necessity . . . you write to save your life.
ALICE WALKER

As many as one in ten women report experiencing trauma around their birth experience. Men report trauma in connection to their experience of birth with similar frequency. In many cases, trauma results from a lack of support needed during the birth process or an unmet fundamental need of the mother or father (see page 278 for a list of birthing women's needs and universal human needs). It can also be the result of overwhelm, shock, pain, fear, disappointment, or other intense sensations or emotions.

Following a traumatic birth, we can feel haunted by intrusive thoughts, feelings, and memories; we may feel numb and disembodied; we may feel an intense desire to share that doesn't feel fully satisfied in speaking to others; we can experience shame, blame, anger, anxiety, depression; or all of it.[7] Birth trauma can make us feel incredibly isolated. In all of these circumstances, writing can help us heal after traumatic birth (in conjunction with additional professional healing support).

Birth Loss

The trauma connected with our births can also be connected to the loss of a pregnancy, the loss of a child. I can't think of much that is more painful than losing a child, whether through abortion, miscarriage, stillbirth, or other loss. For those who have experienced birth loss, writing can give us an opportunity to honor the life we have lost, to grieve fully and without restriction, to remember and thus preserve as much as we can about our truncated time with our child, and so much more. Because the voice of loss is often not given space for expression in our culture, writing can become an important—even vital—venue for our processing.

Writing about birth loss, or any challenging birth experience, is often most nourishing and supportive when approached as a process. Katie began writing her story of loss as a series of journal entries over the course of a few months' time.

Katie, like many survivors of birth loss, was not in the place of creating a single narrative account of her experience. Rather, she wrote her story in manageable pieces as elements came forward for expression and healing.

KATIE'S STORY

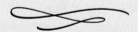

Togetherness

"Togetherness." This is the word Jeremy uses to describe our loss and grief. He always says we are in this together.

"Will we be okay?" I ask him all the time.

"What makes you think we won't?"

He is certain our togetherness is the very medicine we need to get through this.

Since the birth and death of our son, all I've wanted is to be to-gether with Jeremy. I want to sit on our porch with him. I want to lie in bed with him. I want to sit together on the couch with him.

There came a moment in our togetherness, during that four days in the hospital, after our baby was born. We were holding his dead body. And we had to say goodbye.

The nurses stood outside our door while Jeremy, Bambino, and I lay together. Time was weird in the hospital during those four days; it was like being in the airport—a disorienting, new territory trying to locate my luggage, but it was gone—something happened to it, faces I've never seen, a language I've never heard.

Being together with Jeremy and watching our child die together and both of us trying to hold his one-and-a-half-pound body was a difficult, awful, horrible thing. I couldn't look at Jeremy. I remember not even wanting to see his eyes—I didn't want to see this experience mirrored back to me. I couldn't even look at him when I passed Bam-bino to him during his short life.

"Do you want to hold him?"

"Of course."

We both held him while he was alive.

"Here he is," came a disembodied, flat-toned voice, probably the OB when she handed our son—his perfect, beautiful body—to us. In that moment, I didn't, Jeremy didn't, the medical staff didn't know how long Bambino would live.

Jeremy and I—without words, without even looking at each oth-er (because I couldn't)— had to together negotiate how long "long enough" was so that I would pass on our Bambino to Jeremy so he could hold him while he was still alive.

Jeremy and I were together when Bambino came into this world and we were there, together, when his life ended.

"What makes you think we won't be okay?" he says. I start to think, "The same reason we need to stay together."

Urn

The metal holds you, your remains, safely. I am afraid all the time someone will take you. I am worried something will happen to you. I think about how my body couldn't support you but my heart can love you. Can the urn hold you? Protect you?

Blood Moon Eclipse on 9/28/2015

The night he died, there was a blood moon. I was too wrapped up in him to notice: did the sun go in front of the moon or did the moon go in front of the sun?

All I could tell was that sadness eclipsed my vision, my perspective. The whole sky, everything, was washed—no, drenched—in my blood, in my tears. Does grief cycle like the phases of the moon? It feels so. Sometimes my grief is waxing, sometimes waning, and sometimes it is so *full*.

Nights

The salt lamp glows at night. It sits on our dresser, turned on every night. I continue to worry that the bulb will burn out, and Jeremy continues to remind me we have other bulbs.

I still hate going to bed and wondering where my mind will go: four days and three nights in the hospital. The waiting. The hope. The not knowing. The interruptions. The lack of sleep. Not wanting nurses to come into the room. Not wanting the nurses to leave.

"You need your rest," I've been told again and again since last September.

How am I supposed to sleep when dreams of holding our son don't come, but instead: moments of not knowing, being scared, the constant physical checks, the constant beeping of my heart-rate monitor, the constant squeezing of the compression boots, seeing the glare of the hallway's fluorescent lights, feeling so hungry and knowing I couldn't eat, the comments: "You may deliver the baby. The baby may be born alive. The baby will die. How long he or she will live will be very short. He or she might cry. You may need to have a D&C. You can't eat anything."

I couldn't deliver the placenta. Between our son's birth and the decision to go to the OR, I lost blood. A lot of blood. At night, I can still see the nurses taking away large pads of blood and clots and weighing them. I can see Jeremy holding our son's dead body and a bright, glaring light overhead marked a moment and Western medicine had to continue (did I have a choice then?).

At night, I see Jeremy and me pulled apart. This moment was one of many moments when our grief experience would be different; it would be lonely and it would be scary.

The nights are still so hard. My empty body and my empty heart and our empty house. I ask, "Will we be okay?" He says, "What makes you think we won't?"

The Wooden Box

Jeremy made a wooden box from a tree in our yard last winter. His grief made a beautiful container to hold the too many cards and the blanket Bambino was wrapped in the moment he was born. It looks like it could be a coffin for a small child.

It is.

Our Porch

It is a refuge.
A retreat, restorative
Grief in a safe space

Yes.

Jane painted my fingernails

Jane painted my fingernails. Tara bought an air plant. Joyce helped me eat. Three different, strong women acknowledging the unknown and the weight of waiting on the medicine to stop the contractions and dilating. They showed up. They took time. They loved me, Jeremy, and our son. I was taken care of.

Three Weddings

At John and Laura's wedding I was going to be pregnant—showing and pregnant. Instead, less than a month after losing our son, Jeremy and I went to New Hampshire. Without him. I didn't want to go and I didn't want to be there. I still don't know how I could have said, "I don't want to go and I don't want to be there." Jeremy wanted to go. I knew I should go. And didn't know I could say no. Like many things about grief, I couldn't find my voice and I didn't know (and I don't know) how to say, "I don't want to."

I was still bleeding, I cried a lot, and I didn't want to be there.

Like that: a bereaved mother, a bereaved couple.

Pat and Summer's wedding marked two months of loss, of grieving, and of crying. I remember having fun and remember the six of us (sisters and husbands) having a lot of fun together.

I was supposed to be seven months pregnant.

Instead I was a bereaved mother walking the line of wanting everyone to say something like "I'm so sorry" and playing down our grief and lost-ness by directing the focus back to Pat and Summer. Neither really happened and I was empty. I wanted to be the cute pregnant woman at Pat and Summer's wedding, and I wanted our baby at Stef and Vin's wedding. I wanted to be that cute mom, the cute couple with a beautiful, healthy infant. Instead at all three weddings, I was a cautionary tale for young couples, for us, for me.

Expectations

Pregnancies begin with, "I'm/we're going to have a baby," or "We're expecting." When in reality, the phrase should be "I'm/we're going to have a healthy baby," or "We're expecting to carry this baby to full term and we expect the baby to be healthy, vibrant, beautiful." These are the predictions, the working hypothesis I, we, society, the white, middle-to-upper-class culture places on women and couples. It's like making claims:

If I follow every pregnancy book, then my baby will be healthy.

If I don't drink alcohol or eat runny eggs or sushi, then my baby will be healthy.

If I take folic acid before and during pregnancy, my baby will be healthy.

If I make it through the first trimester, I can tell people. I can tell people we're going to have a baby and I made it through the first trimester, so I won't let you down because I will have a healthy baby.

Anne Lamott explains that expectations are resentments waiting to happen. She says, "An expectation is how we expect something to happen that is often based more on desire than fact." Yes. I, we, expected a healthy baby (twice). I expected people to be more supportive during our first year of loss.

Expectation also breeds disappointment. Disappointments were—and are—everywhere: in my heart, my mind, my experiences since January 2015. It was disappointing that I didn't get pregnant two years ago in October 2014—instantly.

Why did I think I would?

What expectations did I place on my mind and our bodies?

When I got pregnant in November 2014, it was easy: I wasn't sick, I felt amazing and I remember thinking how foolish I was to have been upset that I didn't get pregnant in October.

What to Expect When You're Expecting isn't a book I've ever read or talked to anyone about, but I am wondering how my disappointments since January 2015, the month and the year of our first pregnancy loss was, were, will, is, are based on implicit, covert messages like the engaging title of the book *What to Expect When You're Expecting*. And, with the lens of white, Western, middle-to-upper-middle-class female, I look at our losses, specifically birthing a live child and watching him die, and I don't know how not to feel like a failure. (This sounds very dramatic and self-absorbed, but why does the white, middle-to-upper-middle class place so much on power and control and setting expectations?)

Peer Pregnancies

There is sadness, a heart-brokenness, a sense of loss, a sense of comparison, a sense of failure, a shake of identity, a blanket of shame, a shift of self-worth, and a yearning for empathy, connection, and compassion when girlfriends, relatives, and colleagues give birth to healthy, living children after healthy, sustainable pregnancies.

Writing cards and sending gifts seem like an automatic, obligatory response. (Although, in all ways, I want to mark these moments in people's lives. But I wonder if the gift-giving and the card-sending come from the right place. I want to be seen. I want the empathy, the cards, the support, the compassion. . .)

Picking out and shopping for new baby gifts almost mocks and teases me. Resentment rises up when baby shower invites arrive—four? No, five? I've lost count.

How does a bereaved mother set boundaries around baby shower invitations?

How can bereaved parents mark peers' big moments (without comparison? without resentment? without disappointment)?

Can I ask to be seen?

Who do bereaved mothers get be for others?

I want others to show up for me.

But what if I can't show up for others?

Healing Past Traumas

Motherhood as an individual experience is the expression
not only of a biologic process, but also of a psychologic unity
that epitomizes numerous individual memories, wishes, and
fears that have preceded the real experience by many years.
HELENE DEUTCH

There is another type of traumatic birth experience: the kind of birth that brings to the surface buried traumas from our past. Pregnancy and childbirth can activate long-dormant issues from our personal or even collective histories. Psychologists have described how our minds store memories in a sort of filing system of the brain. These are categorized by predominant emotion and magnitude and filed by chronology and impact.

Because birth is such a transitional event that calls us to change on a profound level, it tends to call up some of the more impactful events of our lives, as well as those that had the same emotional nuances of our birth experience, both positive and negative.

Common areas of our past that can be activated during pregnancy and birth include:

- our own birth experience (when we were born);
- our experience with our family of origin, especially our mothers and fathers;
- any major losses we've experienced;
- our sexuality in adolescence and adulthood, including any sexual trauma we may have experienced;
- our body image and relationship with our bodies;
- and our experiences/feelings about love, caring, finances, security, identity, and sexuality.

Consider Rachel Jamison Webster's experiences of past traumas arising during the birth process:

> *Maybe, I thought, I am crying for my own mother, who had not screamed because she'd been alone in her hospital room, spinal tapped and flat on her back when they pulled me out with forceps [. . .] My vagina had been the port of suffering, and in the middle of my labor I remembered it— sexual abuse as a girl, disrespectful sex as an adult, jarring pelvic exams.*
>
> *My own instances of pain began coming at me, but violations I had not experienced firsthand came to me too, in rapid Technicolor flashes. I seemed to be traveling with women through time and place. My mother had been abused, and her mother and hers, and there was an ache at this site as old as the world.*[8]

Facing these old wounds can be painful. Let us also remember that opening these old files in birth can serve us. They present us with an opportunity to heal the past as we heal our births. When we open up these old files, shining the light of awareness on once-buried hurts gives us a chance to rewrite them and to heal the past.

When a woman experiences birth or the times surrounding birth as traumatic and feels that it is linked to the past or some deeper longing that extends beyond the birth, it can be very healing to write about the other major events that feel connected to that birth experience. For example, we might write about our own childhoods and how our parents did or did not care for us. We might write about our experience of a past sexual trauma, which has been inadvertently dredged up by the birth of our child. We might write about our relationship and how our memories of our parents' and other major relationships have surfaced since we became parents.

We might write about whatever is coming up for us—it may not even center around a past event, but a major theme or emotion—such as our sense of security, our deeply held beliefs, our grief around major transitions, our sense of belonging, and so on.

As Claudia Panuthos explains, "When the psychological experience is respected and supported, there is a great opportunity for a mental housecleaning of loss stacks [those files in our minds], and emotional release of historical feelings."[9]

Birth gives us an opportunity, however challenging, to heal old wounds and move forward into the new life that awaits us. (And may I again recommend exploring your past traumas through writing with the support of a qualified care professional.)

Healing What Surrounds Our Birth

Sometimes the trauma of our birth has nothing to do with the birth itself or our undigested past, but about our relationships around the time of our birth—with our partners (or ex-partners), with our parents, with our other children, with friends and family, and with ourselves. Consider how Betsy expresses and works through her relationship with her ex-husband in her story (page 15).

> When aspects of our lives hold trauma, birth can be a pinnacle time of revealing or masking those pains.

Because birth is such a transformative time, honing in on this specific experience can help us access the medicine we need to heal ourselves in other areas of our lives. It is medicine we give ourselves through our writing.

Billy's story of becoming a teen father is a great example of how we process the pain of our lives by writing about our births. Billy has struggled with his relationship with his son's mother since before the birth. As you will see, his birth story is as much the story of a difficult relationship as it is a birth story. Those things—the birth and the relationship—cannot be teased apart: they are inseparable in his mind.

BILLY'S STORY

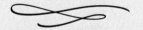

This all starts on a bus ride to Colorado. At the ripe age of fifteen, in my freshman year of high school, my good friend and I signed up for a youth group trip to Colorado to go snowboarding at Steamboat. We could not have been more stoked to take this adventure! Little did I know it would change the entire course of my life. The week before the trip was full of excitement, planning our days, and of course securing a large amount of marijuana and cigarettes to keep us satisfied on the trip. You see, my life was full— full of drugs, board sports, and girls. With little responsibility to keep me down, I took it upon myself to indulge as heavily as I could in all of these things. I was a full-blown addict by the age of fourteen.

Anyway, the day finally came. We started our journey to Steamboat. After several stops, weed breaks and a bottle of Robitussin, I met her. We will call her Lisa. Lisa and some friends were playing a game called Bullshit and Lisa decided I must come play. She would not take no for an answer. I reluctantly agreed. After a while, people faded from the game, and Lisa and I were left to chat. It was the middle of the night. The bus floated along, lulling all but the driver, Lisa, and myself to sleep. Lisa and I did something better than sleep: we had ourselves a make-out session. It was a make-out session that lasted through the trip and for the next year and a half.

I distinctly remember being on the trip around day four, and someone asked if this was just a thing or if this would last after we got back home. That was the first I'd thought about it. I was afraid to admit I wasn't that into Lisa at the time and decided it would be easier to say, "Yeah, totally, it will last."

That's the way I continued to be until about the summer of 1998. After being together for a year of continuous unprotected sex and drugs, I decided it was time to leave Lisa. She was extremely controlling and jealous of every girl in my life, even the ones on TV. Now let me be clear. She wasn't and is not a terrible person. We were just young and stupid. I should have left her long before that, but I was too afraid to hurt her. I had had enough of being treated that way and finally got the cojones to do what I needed to do.

So I finally told her, "I want to break up." That's when it came out.

"I THINK I AM PREGNANT."

I would like to say I was surprised. But I was not. Just plain out afraid. Afraid of what my parents would say, afraid of her parents, afraid of being a dad at what would be seventeen, and afraid to stay with Lisa.

I was so afraid to tell my mother I had my best friend call her at work and break the news. She actually took it pretty well. She wasn't happy, I'll tell you that, but she left the choice to keep the baby, adopt, or abort up to us. My father did as well. He always did well with the really big stuff.

Her parents, however, did not. In the months before, they loved me. They brought me on family trips and always spoke highly of me. However, when we told them, I remember her mother saying, "How could you?" and "We trusted you!" I can fully understand her outrage. I was asked to leave the house.

In the next months, Lisa did everything she could to graduate early. She was a year older than I. She was a senior and I only a junior. Lisa's jealousy got worse, her controlling ways out of control. I was not even allowed to look at the TV when a pretty girl was on, and every girl in school was a suspect. Even talking to one of my five sisters bordered on betrayal to her.

I was a wreck. I was seeing a counselor through all of this. Well, since early summer 1998. The counselor saw I was getting low. Really low. Still heavily self-medicating. I think it was apparent to him something needed to change quickly, and the biggest stressor was being in a relationship I was completely miserable in.

After being advised by my counselor, my mother, my father, and closest friends, I decided to leave her at seven months pregnant.

After speaking to my counselor and others, I concluded that if I knew I was going to leave her, it might as well be now. If things had not been as bad as they were, I don't think that would have been okay, but as an unstable seventeen-year-old drug addict with deep depression, I can give myself empathy.

I just couldn't do it.

I needed a reason to leave so she would never want to be with me.

So I cheated on her.

Now, she didn't know about it, but it added a new layer of toxic shame that couldn't be undone. It was doing her a favor to leave her at that point. I couldn't be loved after that.

I broke the news that I was leaving her over the phone from my father's house. As you can imagine, it did not go well. Not at all. She and our mutual friend drove the hour to pick me up and go for a ride to talk about it. She begged and pleaded. Cried and yelled. I couldn't blame her. But I could not go back.

In the weeks that followed, she went back to smoking pot and cigarettes with no restraint. I went on to harder things like methamphetamines—"crank," we called it—and whatever else I could get my hands on. I began selling drugs again to support my habit.

I was filled with guilt and shame, but at the same time it felt like a great relief! It was really a huge weight off my shoulders. I still wanted to be a huge part of this child's life, and I wanted to be at the birth, and she knew that. She was still very much in love with me and kept me as close as she could. Soon after breaking up, I met a girl. She was beautiful and I fell madly in love with her. That complicated things, as you can imagine. Lisa knew about her. She played it cool for the most part, wanting to keep me close, but I know it tore her apart, further layering this mountain of guilt and shame.

As the due date grew closer, we didn't talk as much. But it was understood that I would be there when he was born. This was very important to me. I may have done some things that objectively seem like terrible things to do. But I am, and have always been, a deep feeler. I really wanted to be there.

On April 16, 1999, I heard word that he was born. I found out where they were and rushed down to the hospital. My dear friend Mark accompanied me; I needed his support. When I arrived at the hospital, Lisa told me it happened very fast and there was no time to call. I was hurt by this but took it as it was. Twenty minutes later her friend, we'll call her Kat, slipped up and mentioned being there for the birth the day before. The stories didn't match up.

Lisa's mother was in the room when I put it all together that Lisa had deceived me and purposely kept me away during the birth of our son. Lisa's mom looked at me and laughed in my face. I became so enraged I needed to leave the room. I had violent tendencies at the time and wasn't sure I could refrain from acting out against Lisa's mother. And after all, she wanted this boy to be aborted and even demanded it, while my parents stood by supportive of Lisa and me in our decision.

I went downstairs to the smoking area and lost it. I was yelling and generally freaking out to Mark. I imagine if it was 2016, I would have been escorted from the property.

Eventually I was able to calm my nerves enough and went back up to the room to see my boy. Regardless of all that had happened with her and me, I was so happy to be his father.

I loved Tanner right away.

I left the hospital that day with so many complex emotions that a seventeen-year-old was not equipped to handle. This resulted in continuous drug use. Lisa followed suit.

Three years passed and we co-parented as best we could. I had him every Monday, Wednesday, and every other weekend and she the opposite days. Things were not perfect with two drug-using parents, but we kept him safe and had help from family.

Eventually Lisa became pregnant again by another guy (her now-husband) in June of 2002. She told me she was moving away to be closer to him in Grand Forks, North Dakota (we grew up in the Twin Cities, Minnesota). I followed shortly after in the month of July 2002. It became apparent right away that her plan was to phase me out. By this point, I had sworn off many of the harder drugs but switched to drinking, which was no better for me, I found.

By January 2003 she told me she was leaving Grand Forks to move farther away to an even more remote town called Middle River, which is in the "middle" of nowhere. I just couldn't go there. I moved back home to the Twin Cities. Lisa moved back for a couple months, and during this time I got to see Tanner several times. I knew she was moving to Middle River soon but not the exact date.

In March, she moved with Tanner, without a trace. She would no longer answer my calls. I had no address. Her parents wouldn't tell me where she was. I was desperate. My using was getting even worse. I was working with friends for cash and living in a camper in my friend's driveway. I knew if I was going to be in my son's life, I needed to get it together.

With help from my father, I got a Rule 25 (an assessment that allowed me to receive public funding for a chemical dependency program) and found myself in treatment for drugs and alcohol. My treatment counselor, Curt, told me: "You only need to change one thing: everything."

Forced to face myself for the first time, I was able to make the drastic life changes I needed to make. After a month of intensive treatment, I went to a halfway house in Duluth and began the year-long journey to get my son back into my life.

To give some closure to this story, I want to share that eventually I did get my son back into my life. By the time I did, he had been told

I was no longer his dad and was just a friend. This tore me to pieces. I stayed strong and continued the high road with his mother, making it a point to pray for her and doing my best to become her friend.

Tanner is seventeen and a senior in high school as I write this. We have a great relationship and enjoy rock climbing, mountain biking, skateboarding, snowboarding, and just hanging out talking together. I have been honest with him about my life, and he is honest with me about his life.

Although his birth didn't go as I wanted it to, we are able to share our lives in a rich, meaningful relationship. I am so grateful for him and all that his birth has brought to me.

He saved my life in so many ways.

He is a pillar of strength for me.

He is my son.

Billy reports that writing about his birth experience—in this case, of not being permitted to be present at all—brought about tremendous awareness, clarity, understanding, and healing:

> The process of writing this has really allowed me to say things that have weighed me down with guilt and shame. Although I have shared these details before with close friends, it is a powerful experience to write it out. It makes it more real to me. Like, There, now it's really out for all to see.

> And now this story—good, bad, or otherwise—is written for my son to read when he is ready, and for my grandkids and theirs. History is often so different than what actually happened. I am so grateful to have this chance to show my kin a bit about who I was through the telling of this birth story.

Seeking Additional Support in Healing Birth Trauma

We all need support through challenging times. Many healing modalities support our full return back into our bodies—bodies that are safe and whole in environments we can learn to trust again—as well as back into our minds, emotions, and spirit.

Movement: Yoga, Qoya (qoya.love)

Somatic Therapies: Somatic Experiencing (somaticexperiencing.com); TRE (tension release exercises; see traumaprevention.com for a list of therapists), "Womb surrounds" (especially good for processing trauma from one's own birth; see castellinotraining.com/process)

Bodywork: Massage, flower essence therapy, craniosacral therapy, Arvigo Techniques of Mayan Abdominal Therapy® and Arvigo® Spiritual Healing

Eye Movement Desensitization and Reprocessing (EMDR): EMDR is considered highly effective in supporting individuals through single incidents of trauma, such as birth trauma.

Mind: Meditation, yoga nidra, psychotherapy

Healing is a journey; we take small but steady steps on its path. I honor you for your bravery and your strength, even if you don't feel brave or strong. Sometimes our hearts break so that they can open. May yours open to something greater than you've ever known before. May your heart, body, mind, and soul heal in time and may you be stronger for having been broken.

CHAPTER SIX

We Write to Honor

ONE OF THE GREATEST REASONS WE WRITE OUR STORIES is to honor them and to honor birth itself. What does it mean to honor something? To honor something is to regard it with great respect, to hold it in high esteem. To honor something is to offer a measure of respect and reverence equal to its worth.

Writing is one way we come into right relationship with birth and with our experiences. Writing is a gesture of humility, of awe, of gratitude, of expressing that which is real and true. When we offer this gesture by committing time and energy to writing the stories that matter most, we naturally come to honor our stories, our experiences, our children, our lives, and birth itself.

When we write, we honor the power of birth. We recognize what birth truly is: the human capacity to create, to bring forth life into this world, to venture with great courage out to that threshold where matter and spirit meet, surrendering to a force much greater than ourselves. We honor what has been honored throughout human history, through all time and space:

that birth is one of the most powerful experiences we'll ever know as humans.

Just look to the hundreds of goddesses of fertility and childbirth that have been venerated throughout time, from Anne (Catholic), Anahit (Armenian), Artemis (Greek), Akna (Inuit and Maya), Atahensic (Iroquois)—and those are just a few of the "A"-named goddesses—all the way to whole teams of holy beings that solely govern birth, including the Chinese Childbirth Monitors of the Nine Heavens and the Hindu Matrikas.

Birth has always mattered deeply and long been held in the reverence it is owed.

When we write, we honor ourselves. We honor that to be a conduit of creation is a massive initiation.

We may never come to a place of celebrating our births, but we can honor them.

We can honor the immensity of our experiences.

We can honor what was and what is.

We honor our own lives, our bodies, hearts, and souls; our courage; our vulnerability; and our love through writing the stories of our births. We can come to a place of really seeing birth for what it is with honest acceptance.

When we write, we also honor our children's lives. We recognize the importance of their beginnings: their personal origin stories. We honor that our birth stories are theirs as much as our own. We pay reverence to the great forces that brought them into the world and into our lives, in whatever shape that took.

Sometimes we don't know how life will call us to honor our births or the lives marked by these monumental beginnings.

Lindsay, whose stories appear below, has found that telling the stories of her sons' births is crucial to her honoring their lives, her mothering, and all that has come with loving Patrick and Logan.

LINDSAY'S STORIES

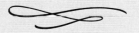

PATRICK CARLYLE MCKINNON
February 12, 2006
Five pounds, Fourteen ounces
4:11 p.m.

Four years after Tom and I had been married, we decided to take our turn seeking new adventures by having a baby. Ravens started showing up everywhere. I mean they were everywhere! It was as though they would follow the car as we ran errands, or, more accurately, they would show us the way. It was amazing how they would swoop down in front and just ahead of the windshield. They would perch on a branch outside our window and do their dance while they called out to others. We would pass apartment complexes and golf courses called Ravenswood and Raven's Peak. The more we noticed and acknowledged them, the more they made themselves known. Funny how that works. I started looking into the meaning and significance of ravens as spirit totems. One morning I was watching *The TODAY Show* and Katie Couric was doing the fashion segment. She asked one of the models what her name was and the model replied, "Raven." In that moment, my body jumped off the couch and grabbed a pregnancy test. A few minutes later it was confirmed: PREGNANT!

Now let me tell you, I am that annoying mom who *loved* being pregnant. I am the mom that other moms rolled their eyes at and want to vomit in response to. My pregnancies were absolutely joyful. I loved every minute of growing my babies. I loved feeling them roll inside of me and stretch into their little beings. I loved sharing the same life-blood and oxygen. I loved listening to them. I loved how my belly felt full of wonder; I felt sexy and radiant; I kept my hands on my belly to feel them, connect with them, and love them through my touch. I was in a constant state of awe and felt the physical abundance that I was privileged to carry.

On Valentine's weekend 2006, thirty-six weeks full, we had a special double date with our close friends Gene and Melonie. We shared a decadent meal at Metro that seemed to last forever. We laughed so hard that *all* of us were grabbing our bellies, not just me! Following dinner, we walked upstairs to the club and danced our asses off. The dance floor has always called my name and I loved feeling Patrick dance inside of me. It was 2:00 in the morning by the time we got home, and Tom and I fell into bed, exhausted and on cloud nine. But not for long. . .

My first contractions woke me up shortly after 3:00 in the morning. At first I tried to ignore them but they persisted. I pulled myself out of bed and shuffled downstairs to the couch in the living room. Our dogs Zeke, a blue-eyed Siberian Husky, and Sydney, a blue merle Australian Shepherd, followed me. For the first hours of labor, they were my doulas. I didn't want to wake up Tom yet, not until I knew that I was in active labor. Zeke stood guard for me, in the room but with his back turned and facing the door. Sydney was right beside me, resting her head on the pillow with mine as I breathed through each contraction, stroked her ears, and drifted into sleep between each wave. Her eyes reassured mine as the contractions increased in frequency and intensity. Animals get it. Animals get all things natural, and having a baby was no different.

Eventually I moved from the couch to leaning over the kitchen counter, rocking and swaying from side to side, moving through each surge and softening my entire being. I woke Tom up around 7:00 a.m.

"What do you want me to do?" he asked.

"Keep sleeping for now, I'll need your energy later. But know that today is the day."

He always has perfect timing and joined me a little while later with a cup of coffee. Contractions were getting harder, and I needed him to apply pressure to my lower back for relief. We continued swaying, groaning, touching, breathing, kissing, softening, melting, surrendering to the direction in which my body wanted to take me. I did not hold on to anything. Holding on to contractions makes them more painful.

We called our midwife, Wanda Smith, who answered the phone in a whisper.

"Wanda, I need you to come over. I'm in labor, and Patrick is ready to go."

"Okay, Baby," she whispered, "You could be in labor for a long time. I'm in church right now and will come over to check you after the service."

"Wanda, Jesus wants you *here*."

It wasn't long before she was at our front door with her entire family in the van. Yes, she confirmed I was in active labor, and she would be back after she dropped her family at home, picked up her midwifery bag, and called her assistant, Crystal. Besides, "a watched pot never boils," she said. Meanwhile, Tom called our friends Rob and Jessica and Gene and Melonie to come over. We were supposed to have a Valentine's lunch with Rob and Jessica, and clearly we were shifting to Plan B. Luckily, Jessica had recently finished her first round in med school on the labor and delivery floor. Hospital birth and home birth are quite a bit different, so she was ripe for learning, and I certainly appreciated her support and knowledge nonetheless.

They brought us the birth tub, an inflatable baby pool from Toys R Us, and set it up in the dining room and began filling it with warm water: 98 degrees to reflect the temperature in the womb, to soften the cervix and to relieve contractions. They also stuffed our fridge with delicious food. Their son, Riley, was about seven years old, and he came into our bedroom, wide-eyed. His eyes were magnetized to my belly. As I lay on my bed, I let him place his hand on my belly so he could feel a contraction.

"Are you okay?" he asked.

"I am more than okay. I am having a baby, and he is going to be here soon." His blue eyes took it all in and his shoulders dropped.

On the next contraction, my water broke with a gush. "Umm, Riley? Can you go get Tom for me, please?"

Gene and Melonie are acupuncturists, and I wanted to leverage the benefits of acupuncture to further ease my contractions. Melonie operated in stealth mode, needling me and giving me herbs through-out labor in a way that was cat-like and precise. Wanda and Crystal showed up and IT. WAS. ON. Everyone had a role and played it beau-tifully. I was able to focus on each contraction with peace and shifted into my zone. . .that zone where every woman goes in order to bring forth life.

In the mid-afternoon, Wanda checked my cervix while I was in the tub and asked me if I was ready to greet my baby boy. I was fully dilated and he was just choosing his time. We got out of the birth tub and walked up the stairs with a few more intense contractions on the way. I leaned into Tom, and we eventually made it to our bed. I took a few contractions on hands and knees, and then I flipped to my side. Wanda called for Tom's assistance (he and Jessica had been fumbling with the video camera), and in the calmest and most grounding de-meanor, she taught him exactly what to do. He was dialed in and focused like I've never seen before.

With each contraction, you could see Patrick's wrinkled pink head easing through, a little more each time. I looked into Crystal's loving eyes as my body spontaneously bore down, pushing through the "ring of fire" where a woman stretches to her peak. It burned. Oh my God, it burned, but I didn't care. On the next contraction, Patrick bolted through me like a rocket, and Tom literally lunged across the bed and caught his first-born child in his own two hands. What a holy moment. What an intense and joyful moment! All of us burst into laughter, and then, in complete awe, were rendered silent. There was celebration and my Baby Boy was here.

Eventually, directed by our midwife, Tom cut the cord, and Pat-rick, my Valentine, snuggled on my chest, all glorious and gooey and wet and absolutely beautiful. I fell in love all over again in that mo-ment. I had found my purpose, and was happier than ever.

The moments that followed his birth were a little hectic, but I was happy to be at home, in my own space, my own comfort zone, my own privacy, my own everything. We weighed Patrick and measured him right there on the bed. The midwives did their newborn checks, and all ten toes and fingers were kissed and accounted for. We wiped the vernix from his body and giggled at the feel of his soft baby bottom. He was so small! Our friends cooked a delicious warm meal and we toasted his birth with mimosas before settling into a lifetime of snuggles and learning how to navigate each new chapter.

LOGAN HAYES MCKINNON
April 15, 2010
six pounds, seven ounces
3:01 a.m.

I was feeling that pull again. You know, that visceral pull that can make a woman crazy because she wants a baby so badly? There is no compromising with a woman desiring a baby. Hormones took over, and I was not myself. There was an underlying anxiety that I could not control. I received regular acupuncture to help calm and prepare my body. I prayed harder than ever and pleaded with the moon. I took my temperature every morning and charted my cycles. I pounced on Tom every time I ovulated with a ferocity that was, well, not so sexy. With each passing month, I grew more frustrated and emotional as pregnancy tests showed up negative.

My birthday was coming up, and I wanted to escape and get out of town. Our friend, River, and his world fusion jazz band, was playing in Black Mountain, North Carolina, just four hours from where we live in Roanoke, Virginia. Mariam, a heaven-sent Armenian vocalist, was singing with them at this concert, and everything in my body wanted to be bathed in that sound. I begged Tom to take me— you know, for "my birthday." It worked.

When we showed up at the concert, Mariam was ripe with pregnancy and absolutely glowing. My heart pounded and jumped into my throat. I had no idea she was pregnant! As we danced to River's drum and she took the stage, she channeled the heavens with her voice and called in Spirit. I could feel it, everywhere.

Goosebumps covered my body, and tears swelled and rolled down my cheeks. I was absolutely mesmerized by her voice and movement as she gently stroked her beautiful belly and sang in her traditional language. I had no idea what she was saying, but I just knew it was for me. I was captivated, moved, inspired, and rendered in awe. That night, Tom and I happened to stay in a hotel in Asheville—the same hotel where we hosted our epic wedding reception years ago. Our child was conceived that beautiful night.

It wasn't too long after that night in Asheville when Patrick, almost four, and I had been playing at the park. I even remember what I was wearing: my purple Patagonia Margot dress, Chacos, and my yellow "Life Is Good" ball cap. After a day of sliding, swinging, and creeking, I loaded him with his sun-kissed face into the truck, and we headed home.

On the way up the driveway, I slammed on the breaks. There was a turtle in the middle of the driveway. I put the truck in park and got Patrick out of his car seat. We picked up that amazing turtle and Patrick noticed the colors and counted the sections of his shell, each section for the number of moons in the calendar year. I asked my little shaman what this could possibly mean. But I already had a sense. Again, goosebumps. I shuffled Patrick inside the house and reached for a pregnancy test. PREGNANT! All smiles and then some! I gifted Tom with the pregnancy tests confirming the fact that we were positively committed to yet another grand adventure into parenthood.

Days later at another park, Patrick played with his friends Maggie and Carter. Their mom, Amber, greeted me with a hug. "Oh my God, you are glowing. Are you pregnant? You ARE pregnant, I can tell." The secret was out.

That winter went by all too quickly. I loved being pregnant in the wintertime. April approached, and my sister Clarissa shared with me that having a baby on her birthday would be the best present ever.

She got her wish. Of course, there is always a challenge before every birth, and ours was the plumbing in our house. This time, it was the master bathtub upstairs that leaked through the floors downstairs and damaged the walls and ceiling, etc., etc. Tom worked his tail off at work that week and came home to replace sheetrock and spackle our walls. He was exhausted. He was also keenly aware.

Tom knew I was in labor, though I held my tongue and did not say a word. I just breathed and moved through the contractions and continued with the tasks at hand. It was just before Patrick's bedtime and I wanted to savor every moment I had with him. I knew that as soon as I gave in to my body, I would no longer be a mom of one, but two Light Beings.

Patrick had extra time in the bath, and I savored the moments of splashing and washing his hair. I read extra stories to him at bedtime, sang a few more songs than I usually do, and prayed a little longer, choosing my words very carefully. I cried as I hugged and kissed him good night, knowing that his world was about to change forever. I wanted him to love his little brother and love him fiercely. I wished for them to be best friends and for Patrick to be the most loving big brother. And why would I think anything otherwise? Patrick LOVED my baby belly! He loved hugging and kissing my belly, talking to his brother though the womb, and reading stories to him. Patrick also loved massaging my belly, and his touch was always gentle and caring. He knew his little brother in utero as well as Tom and I did. Contractions grew stronger, and I had to peel myself away from him that night.

I was ready for the next chapter, but was I really?

As soon as I walked downstairs, I heard Tom snap the stepladder shut. With the household project officially complete and Patrick down to sleep, we could focus 100 percent on the next chapter at hand. At this point, we knew it was a boy and had spoken about names but I had surrendered the decision to Tom months ago. It is difficult to come up with the perfect name sometimes. We narrowed it down to five possible names, and I asked Tom to discuss them with

Patrick and choose. I wanted Tom to introduce me to our son as I held him in my arms for the first time.

We were planning another home birth, this time a proper water birth with the Cadillac of all birth pools set up in my massage studio. My friend Melinda was to be our doula and, of course, Wanda and Crystal were back for round two. Crystal also happened to be pregnant and due any day, and we weren't sure if she would be able to show up or not.

I ended up having my baby on Crystal's due date. Contractions brought me to my knees. Holy fuck, they were intense! This one was *not* like the first time! This baby gave no warning or warm-up, and it was a huge challenge to stay on top of the contractions and not let them overwhelm or get away from me. Though I tried, I could not stand or lean over a counter as I had with Patrick. This one brought me to the floor on my hands and knees with every single contraction. The sensations quickly reached from my low back to my groin, over my belly and down through the insides of my legs to my feet. It took all of me to navigate the pain and pressure. I could not speak.

Tom had called our birth team and set them all in motion. On the periphery of my zone, I heard them all show up one by one, and then I heard Crystal's voice. She made it! Her voice in particular relaxed any anxiety I was feeling about whether or not I could handle this. Beyond a shadow of a doubt, I knew I could handle anything. I labored in the guest room downstairs until I heard Wanda tell me I was six centimeters dilated and ready to get in the birth tub. What music to my ears! Before six centimeters, a birth pool will slow down the labor. After six centimeters, it will speed it up and provide as much relief from the pressure as an epidural would in the hospital. I dropped my jaw when I opened the door to the massage room where everything was set up. It was a sensual sanctuary.

Candlelight and rose petals adorned every surface, everywhere. Statues of goddesses graced the corners of the room. Music was playing. Essential oils were spritzed about. Melinda stood in the middle of the room and with a single motion of her hand, she invited me into my warm birth tub which was also adorned with rose petals and floating candles. It was a holy space, and one made with the specific intention and prayers to bring my baby into this world. The water was warm, and I fully immersed my body. My contractions immediately responded, and it was as though my baby took a sigh of relief with me. I floated from birth position to birth position and could feel him move inside of me, as well. I fell back into the arms of my husband.

I was completely and totally embodied in my most sensual self, all six senses heightened in their fullest power, channeled, and purpose-driven. I felt every breath, in and out. I felt like a goddess, and I knew I had called this all in. I was a vessel of divine strength and Love. I trusted my body, and I trusted my baby. Goodness, he was strong and he wanted to go fast, but I worked with him to slow him down, just a little bit. I met my baby's surges with my breath and hip circles and asked him to go easy on his mama. I felt pressure in my womb and pelvis. The pain I felt on the outside of this water sanctuary had been diffused. I was buoyant and light, relaxed, and in my zone. I welcomed every sensation into my being and rode it through my body as though I was surfing the ocean waves with ease and grace. I prayed and spoke to my baby, letting him know we were on his time, and he was leading the way.

Tom was in the birth pool with me. "All ten Toms" came into complete focus and were holding space for me, for our baby. My eyes were closed, but I could feel him studying my face and my every expression. He was not going anywhere and was ready whenever we were ready. Wanda and Crystal could see the baby's head come through and were amazed that even in the water, his eyes were open and ready for the world! They shined a flashlight through the water so we could also see. He was *there*. He was ready, but wait. . . I clamped down and held him tighter in my womb. I remember thinking that my life—our life—would never be the same. Although I was excited about the future and what a family of four would bring, I wanted to honor our one last moment.

Crystal must have read my mind because I heard her say, "It's okay, Lindsay, you can let go now and let him come through." Sometimes that's all women need: permission from another woman to gain the strength to do the next right thing. On the following breath and contraction, I looked Tom in the eyes and said, "I love you," just as my body bore down and completely surrendered. Our baby Boy exited my body, slithering his body out, and floating into the warm water that mirrored my womb. Without gravity, and with much more room to expand, he unfolded his own arms and legs gently and gracefully and swam his way to the top, where the water met the air. In that instant, Tom swept him up, and our baby boy took his first breath. Tears streamed down all of our faces and he wiggled his way onto my chest.

"Oh my God, Baby, you did it," Tom said.

We all welcomed this turtle-bug into being and huddled together in the pool, smothering him with kisses. I wish I could go back to that moment right there. It was magical.

Outside the tub, and sitting on the birth stool, we covered him with warm blankets and wiped the vernix off his little body. Tom embraced the both of us from behind and for the first time, called him by name, "Hello, Logan. Welcome to our world. We've been waiting for you." I gasped and sank even further into my exploding heart. Yes . . . Logan. Logan is his name! Logan Hayes McKinnon... I repeated his name over and over again.

Logan was born at 3:01 in the morning on April 15. Again, all the newborn exams took place right there on the bed with the careful supervision of both dogs, Sydney and Zeke, and we relaxed into being parents all over again. Logan was weighed and measured. He was a natural at nursing, and we were in awe of that soft baby butt. Around 7:00 in the morning, Tom went upstairs to wake up Patrick and share the good news.

Tom: "Good morning Buddy. I have a surprise for you."
Patrick: "What is it?"
Tom: "How about you guess."

Patrick: "Umm. . . a robot or something?"

Tom: "No, not quite. Guess again."

Patrick: "Illuminator light-up running shoes?"

Tom: "Nope. That's not it either. Guess again."

Patrick: "A Transformer? I'm all out of guesses."

Tom: "What if I told you that last night while you were sleeping, your baby brother was born."

Patrick: "He's HERE?"

Tom: "Wanna go meet him?"

Patrick: "Sure."

Tom: "Are you nervous?"

Patrick: "No."

Tom: "Excited?"

Patrick: "YES!"

Tom carried Patrick, then four years old, downstairs. As they arrived at the bedroom door, he insisted on walking in by himself. He leapt up on the bed and crawled over to me and Logan, rubbing and patting his back, cupping his head and gazing into the eyes of this his baby brother with the biggest smile on his face. In the gentle enthusiasm with which he responded to his baby brother, I knew Patrick had found his purpose, as well. He wanted to hold him, hug him, and kiss him. We spent all day playing and snuggling together as a family of four.

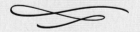

My children were born at home, and they died at home.

They were born in water. They died in a tragic house fire in March 2016. Patrick was ten, and Logan was just a few weeks shy of turning six.

To write their story, which is also mine, is cathartic, and healing, and filled with emotion and longing. I had written their birth stories soon after their births, but of course lost those pieces in our house fire that took everything. Claiming their birth stories means that they were in fact living and breathing on this earth. To come to the keys and to rewrite their birth stories post-fire has been even more cathartic, healing, emotional, and filled with longing than before, as I open myself to feel all of it more deeply in my heart, in my body, and in my soul. Writing their story helps me to grieve, and grieving is a good and healthy thing to do.

Sharing their stories helps to celebrate and honor their very important, adventurous lives. Sharing their stories celebrates and honors mine, and what I have created, and what I have been through. Maybe it also gives another woman permission to feel that much more. Maybe it also points the way for someone else. Maybe it helps another human being realize that they are not alone in what they are creating, or going through, and to honor that knowledge as wisdom.

And synchronicity does not fall short on me. As I write these words, my own mother is driving into town to celebrate what would have been Logan's seventh birthday this weekend. There is no coincidence here. How we birth matters. Sharing those birth stories is essential to our shared humanity and humanness.

The impact our boys have had on the lives of others in their short years is immeasurable. They loved, and they loved big. We grow up hearing the words, "Nothing separates us from the love of God." I have learned the hard way that there is nothing truer than these words. Patrick and Logan continue to reach out across any physical limitations and break through the realms of the Divine to express their love to each and every one of us, daily. They have infused their love into *everything*, everywhere. They have fully embodied Love in every sense of that word, and still, like that raven years ago, they show us the way. More than anything on earth, I miss holding them and snuggling them, watching them grow and change. I still feel their love but not their physical touch, and that is the hardest part to navigate. It is with this sentiment that I ask each and every one of you to reach out physically to your loved ones and touch them; honor that sensation of physical touch that we are gifted with, and let them know how much you love them. Don't waste a second resisting this gift to love and be loved by another human being.

To moms with Earth Angels and moms with Heavenly Angels. To women who are becoming moms and to women who want to be moms. To all of those who have lost their moms, and to all the moms who grieve the loss of their children and continue to love them from across The Veil. May we all come back to Love and dare to birth that Love into our world.

CHAPTER SEVEN

Fathers' and Partners' Stories

*U*NTIL RATHER RECENTLY, perhaps the last fifty to sixty years, fathers routinely dwelled on the periphery of birth, which was traditionally the exclusive domain of women. In the late 1800s, for example, when most babies were born at home, it was an unquestioned assumption that men would take no part in their partners' births. They may have been given some ancillary practical task, such as boiling water, but they were not expected, or really even allowed, in the birthing mother's inner circle of support.

Beginning around the late 1940s across many industrialized nations, both men and women increasingly desired fathers' close physical proximity to their birthing partners during labor and birth. In the '50s and '60s, fathers progressively moved from waiting room to bedside, acting as coaches to their birthing partners through labor and birth. Men became increasingly involved in the creative process of pregnancy and birth—beyond the sexual act—and adopted more and more of a nurturing role, first with their partners and then with their children. In 1975, for example, fathers spent just 15 minutes with their child(ren) each day, and in the late '90s, that number had increased eightfold.[8]

Today in the Western world, some ninety percent of all fathers are present at the birth of their children.[9] It is almost absurd these days to question whether or not Dad should be present at his child's birth. Presently, we expect a lot out of our male companions at birth. Some of us rely almost exclusively on their support as we birth our babies. During pregnancy, we expect our expectant fathers to attend childbirth classes, attend prenatal appointments, and read books on birth and fatherhood. This is all new territory for men, evolutionarily speaking.

Participating in labor, witnessing birth, and holding their newborn babies have a profound effect on fathers physiologically, psychologically, and spiritually.

Research has shown that hormonal activity is altered in men during their partner's pregnancy.[10] These hormonal effects are even more dramatic when Papa attends the birth. These chemical messengers—namely prolactin, oxytocin, and vasopressin—are all higher than normal in men around the time of birth. Each of these hormones plays a role that supports the father in nurturing and caring for his partner and child. The increased prolactin promotes bonding, attachment, and caring. The increased oxytocin kick-starts his paternal nurturing instincts. The increased vasopressin compels a man to protect his family and remain loyal to them. It seems that it is not just culture that supports fathers' presence at birth—Mother Nature herself offers him a chemical toolkit to foster his close involvement in pregnancy, birth, and early parenting.

Studies have found that a father's presence in the immediate postpartum period influences him profoundly. One study of Israeli fathers, for example, found that after just seven hours with their newborn children, each father could reliably identify his child while blindfolded just by touching his baby's hands. Just as the mother does, the father changes the pattern and pitch of his voice instinctively in correspondence to baby's signals in the early postpartum period.[11]

In addition to influencing their physiology, birth affects men on a profound psychological level. Virtually all fathers report that the experience of witnessing their partner give birth has a dramatic effect on their identities, their relationships to their partners, and their relationships to their children. When a father experiences birth positively, he tends to feel as if he already has a relationship with the child, feels more comfortable holding his child, and feels more confident in his parenting abilities in the postpartum period.

For many fathers, birth can also be experienced as a shock to the system, one that requires processing and integration. For this reason, birth story writing can be a crucial tool of the new father, just as it is for the new mother.

In their birth stories, many contemporary fathers express an intense desire—often coupled with anxiety—to perform up to the expectations of their partners and those around them during the birth experience. Many have a deep desire to "do it right." Being oriented toward action and solutions, many men want to *do* the right thing and are afraid of *doing* the wrong thing. One secret they may come to discover is that their *being* is actually ninety percent of their role through birth and labor. Who you *are* and your *presence* are far more important than what you *say* or *do*. Men who are able to provide stability, attentiveness, and responsiveness by their mere presence offer their partners a profound level of support. This is called holding space. We offer ourselves and our energy as a container to hold steady, to anchor and ground, as our beloved women move powerfully though the peaks and valleys, surges and seismic shifts of their birth adventure.

This holding space requires a great degree of relinquishing control, one of the great lessons of birth for both men and women. Surrendering control can be quite difficult for a man accustomed to having a good degree of control in his life (same goes for women). Facing the feminine realm of birth—which moves not linearly, logically, or predictably—can turn the world upside down for anyone (man or woman), who dwells mostly in the tidy, orderly masculine realm.

Some men may feel overwhelmed and underprepared for what is required of them, both practically and intangibly, as they move through their own intense and changing inner landscapes in birth. For some, profound fear may arise—fear over the safety of their partner or of their child, fear of disappointing their partner, fear of not being up to the task of partnering and parenting. Some are bewildered by the hospital environment and their place in it; some are unclear whether what their partner is experiencing is normal and feel overwhelmed by the decisions they are asked to make as the birth process unfolds.

Lance's story shows an internal landscape common to many men as they make their way through the birth experience—an assessment of their own preparedness, their need to adequately support their partners, their desire to get fathering "right" from the start, and the magnitude of one's transformation into a dad.

LANCE'S STORY

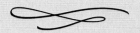

My wife jolted me out of a deep sleep at 5:00 a.m. She mumbled something didn't "feel right." The fear in her voice scared me.

I slowly followed her into the bathroom.

"Something feels wet," she replied. She wondered aloud, "Did my water break? I thought there's supposed to be a pool of water on the floor. That's what it's always like on TV." Within minutes we were in a taxi headed to the hospital.

After the battery of tests, the doctor confirmed my wife's suspicions, then ordered an emergency C-section within the hour.

At this moment, life froze and an incredible sense of calm washed over me. Like an athlete pumping himself up for a playoff game, I took my wife's hand and said, "We need to mentally prepare for what's about to happen. We are going to go through this together."

My failures to prepare for this moment immediately flashed through my mind: We didn't pack a bag for the hospital, the car seat was still in the box, the furniture for the nursery wouldn't be delivered for two weeks, I never cracked a page in any of the parenting books stacked on my shelf, and I never glanced at the websites recommended by the veteran dads. If there were an expectant dad exam, I'd have scored a zero. Perhaps it was this shocking realization that somehow numbed me into conveying the calm and collected demeanor my wife needed upon learning our baby would be born today—a month earlier than expected.

Before long, I was donning a pair of scrubs in the delivery room. All the while, I was clenching my wife's hand, kissing her forehead, and whispering confidently about how we were going to be such amazing parents.

A pause. A commotion. I saw the doctor whisk our son over to a team of nurses.

I locked on my wife's eyes. "Where was the cry? Is everything all right?" she said. The seconds felt like hours. Finally, a blissful, shrieking cry.

We were parents! I was a dad!

My own first twenty-four hours of fatherhood became a comedy of errors.

Wanting to be an engaged father, I was anxious to get some hands-on training while my wife observed from her hospital bed. I slowly unhinged his diaper and removed it before lining up the new one. That cost me big time! A stream of pee shot my way and onto my shirt. My wife and I were hysterical with laughter. Is this what parenting was going to be? Would we live by the mantra, "The one who can laugh at himself will never cease to be amused?"

Our birthing class instructor stressed becoming a "swaddle master" because babies loved that snug feeling that only a tightly wrapped blanket can provide. I reached into our baby supply cart and started fluffing and folding the blanket for my first swaddle. I mummified our newborn. Pieces of blanket stuck out in odd places. The wrap was loose. This was, suffice it to say, oddly challenging work. I called a nurse for guidance and she whipped our son into a perfect cocoon. I felt small. Wasn't there a way to do this more easily with duct tape or with Velcro?

The nurse gave me verbal instructions that sounded simple, so I headed to the nursing lounge because I believed the warm and inviting setting would foster success. I tried to put the bottle's nipple on his lips, and nothing happened. "Does it smell right? Why won't his lips latch on? Am I holding him properly?" After twenty frustrating minutes, I brought our son to the nurses' station and asked for help.

Bottom line: The first day of fatherhood is a humbling experience—not to mention a blow to the ego. I found myself quickly outside my comfort zone and not very good at addressing our son's needs. Consequently, I understood that with any new job, there exists a learning curve. You've got to get into the trenches, practice, and follow your gut instincts. Most importantly, I established a positive partnership with my wife from the get-go and found how much easier parenting can be when we help each other and share in the responsibility.

I suppose above all I'm glad to have been granted those first twenty-four hours to begin with—trial and error included.

While we've so far focused on a father's experience of birth, a same-sex partner present at the birth of their child (or partners, if they are adopting a newborn) has a profoundly transformative experience just like any other, yet also in a unique way. At present, this is a more marginalized voice in our cultural conversation about birth, and it comes with its own complexities. I believe the parts of these stories that are unique to their authors are important to see and honor, as well as the parts that are shared by all those who give or experience birth. We'll see just one example of this in Jason's story below.

All partners have powerful and important experiences of birth, and they have valuable birth stories worth writing.

I encourage fathers and partners to use the information, exercises and prompts in this book, nearly all of which apply to anyone moved to write a birth story.

JASON'S STORY

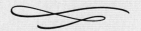

Background

My partner Brandon and I are a gay couple in Utah, and we'd always wanted to grow our family. We already had four girls through my partner's previous marriage, but I'd always wanted to have "my own" kids and to be able to develop and experience that kinship bond firsthand. Despite some initial reservations, I was finally able to talk Brandon into a fifth child. Long story short, we decided on a surrogacy agency in Oregon, one of the few states with pretty relaxed laws with regard to surrogacy. Utah at the time did not allow same-sex couples to use surrogates (and probably still doesn't).

As part of the sign-up process, Brandon and I created a one-page biography about ourselves and our family that the agency could share with potential surrogates. After waiting about three months, we got our first match. We scheduled a Skype call so we could meet "face-to-face," as easy as face-to-face can be given that we are 600 miles from Oregon. In the one-hour call, we not only shared our stories, but it seemed like we became instant friends. Brandon and I knew we'd hang out with Scarlett and her husband if they lived nearby. Since we were conducting the call at home, they met not only us, but also

Emerson, our youngest daughter, who was three at the time, and our two dogs. I remember getting off the call with Brandon, and both of us knowing in our hearts that they were the ones who would help us realize our dreams. They are a down-to-earth couple with two beautiful kids, and we could tell they really wanted to help a family grow. Thankfully, they felt the same way.

Surrogacy in a Nutshell

There are two main types of surrogacy: traditional surrogacy, where the surrogate is also the biological parent, and gestational surrogacy, where the egg donor and the surrogate are two different women. We opted to go the gestational surrogacy route, which is the most common form of surrogacy. The surrogacy process is subject to some very strict requirements and involves a lot of testing; medications for both the egg donor and surrogate; psychological evaluations, including of us, to make sure we're fit parents; and doctor's visits. Since we wanted to improve our chances of a successful surrogacy, both the donor and I were tested for myriad genetic disorders. Fortunately, neither of us is predisposed to any hereditary diseases.

Because of these strict requirements, we were required to create embryos, freeze them, and conduct an embryo transfer when Scarlett was ready. We also conducted some genetic testing of our embryos and found out we could choose whether to transfer a boy or a girl. While it's usually frowned upon, the medical clinic let us choose because we already have four girls; they call it gender balancing. The girls were excited too. . . Kate, who was seven at the time, made it a point to let us know she did not want another sister!

The Process Begins

With the time it took to create embryos and the plan to avoid late pregnancy during the summer, everything worked out for a mid-August embryo transfer. This was our second try, so the anxiety and fear of an unsuccessful transfer was on everyone's minds. Scarlett was just as anxious as we were to find out whether the transfer was successful, so she did a few pregnancy tests at home before her first official pregnancy test, and each time, the pink strip got darker and darker. . . we knew we were pregnant! When we got to the third set of doctor's visits and the second trimester, our worries started to wane, and the fertility clinic was ready to hand Scarlett off to her primary care physician.

As this was my first time going through the process, each step and benchmark was new and exciting. Thankfully, Brandon was there each step of the way to explain what was going on. He even pulled out one of his med school anatomy books after the embryo transfer to give me a refresher on how everything was supposed to work. There is nothing like a home maturation course between two gay men.

Anyway, nine months seemed like a long way away. We couldn't wait for Alex to arrive.

One unique aspect about surrogacy is that everything is planned; you even have a more accurate due date, since the process involves transferring a five-day-old embryo. Everything, that is, except the day the baby wants to arrive. Our son Alex was due on May 3, 2014, so I'd planned on flying up to Oregon on April 21 to spend the last couple of weeks with Scarlett and her family. She'd been doing a great job of sending us pictures and videos of her belly (much to the chagrin of our teenager, who thought that AJ's kicking and moving around was "gross"). Brandon and I thought it was hilarious and a good way to promote abstinence! Anyway, I was excited to be able to experience it in person rather than just seeing her pregnancy pictures and videos.

It was Easter evening, April 20, and Brandon's family had just thrown us our third baby shower when labor began. We got a text from Scarlett at around 8:00 that night letting us know that her water had broken. I'd already packed for my flight out the next evening, but I'd really wanted to be at the birth. As it was already pretty late in the evening, there were no flights out that night, and my flight the next day wasn't going to get me there in time. We tried our hardest to find flights in the morning, but the airline's website kept crashing on us.

Brandon, in his excitement, suggested, "What the hell, let's drive." My first reaction was "Really?! We don't even know how long that's going to take us." Driving had never crossed our minds, and driving in the middle of the night didn't sound sane to me, especially since we'd be up all night, but I mapped it, and we could be in Portland in less than eleven hours. We looked at each other, both realizing that our options were pretty limited, so we shrugged our shoulders and said, "Let's do it!"

I couldn't believe that we were going to hop in the car, with no notice, and drive 600 miles to meet our son. I was dreading the drive but felt like a giddy little schoolgirl, excited that we were about to welcome our son to the world.

Once we got on the road, I started to grill Brandon with questions: "What does it mean that her water broke? How long does it usually take after her water breaks?" and so on. Thankfully, Brandon was patient and filled me in on all the details, including letting me know that her water breaking didn't necessarily mean that she'd have the baby anytime soon; he cautioned that it could be a while. Although her water had broken earlier in the evening, Scarlett didn't head to the hospital until about 2:00 a.m. At that point, we were a little less than halfway to Oregon. According to Google Maps, we weren't due to arrive in Oregon until about 7:00. Scarlett's contractions were pretty steady, so we knew we'd have time. We touched base with Scarlett right outside Portland, and she didn't have much to report and told us to go ahead and head to the hotel to get cleaned up. She assured us we had plenty of time.

For her day job, outside of being a mother of two, Scarlett has her own business as a doula. Given her experience, she was definitely a wealth of knowledge. She was constantly sending us news articles and studies and had even helped us create a birth plan for the hospital. She not only helped me learn a lot, but she also was able to teach Brandon a thing or two (but he'd never admit to it). Anyway, when we got to the hospital, the first people we met were Scarlett's doula, a doula-in-training, and Scarlett's business partner, who is also a doula. With Brandon's training as a doctor, Scarlett's experience, and three doulas, I knew we were in good hands!

When we got to Portland, I called my sister to give her the news. She was excited for us, albeit a little anxious that I was about to be responsible for a newborn. The excitement and probably a bit of anxiety prompted her to ask if I wanted her to be in Portland with us. She'd researched flight options and could be in Portland by 5:00 p.m. With a newborn, I knew we could use the extra help, so I told her to get up there.

We waited for a few hours at the hospital, but labor wasn't progressing. Scarlett knew her body and told us to go get some sleep. At that point, we'd been up for nearly thirty hours. She said she'd keep us posted. We slept, my sister arrived, and we got to spend some quality time with Scarlett, her husband, and her friends, but AJ wasn't in a hurry. By around 6:00 p.m., the doctors were starting to pressure Scarlett on antibiotics and other medicines to move the process along, but she wasn't having any of it. She wanted a natural birth and didn't want anything for the baby that would cause him any potential side effects. As she'd had her two kids at home, the hospital environment was probably the main reason the labor wasn't progressing. Scarlett finally kicked all of us out of her room so she could spend some time with her husband and focus on having our baby.

It worked!

At around 8:45 p.m., Scarlett was in active labor. My sister, Brandon, and I were in the waiting area when we got the call to join the birth. As Brandon and I were walking to her room, we could hear a scream. At first I thought Alex had arrived, but no, it was Scarlett. As a man who had never experienced a birth, I was honestly a bit overwhelmed. As we walked into the room, Kristy (Scarlett's business partner and best friend) saw the "deer in headlights" look on my face and grabbed my arm to reassure me that this was all normal. We were lucky to be surrounded by such amazing people.

The whole birth process seemed to flash before my eyes. Since Scarlett had already been in active labor by the time we got back there, it didn't take long before Alex's head started to appear. The entire experience seemed so surreal. I knew we were going to have a baby, we'd planned for it, but being there for the actual birth still seemed unreal. I don't know if it was adrenaline or the lack of sleep, but everything seemed to move so fast. Once Alex started to appear, the active pushing seemed to last only minutes. He was finally here! The reality of it still hadn't sunk in, everything was moving so fast. Next thing I knew, the doctor handed Alex to Scarlett, and someone was handing me a clamp and scissors. As nervous as I already was, Brandon wasn't helping. I could hear in the background him joking about not cutting off the baby's penis. Fortunately, it didn't happen. While I was a bit overwhelmed, being able to take part in Alex's birth was one of the most memorable and precious experiences of my entire life.

As the doctors and nurses were moving Scarlett to her bed, Kristy told me to take off my shirt and sit down, so I could hold Alex and get in some skin-to-skin bonding time. I'm not sure what the skin-to-skin time does for babies, but I will never forget the feeling as I held our son for the first time. The reality that we were new parents was finally sinking in, and words can't describe how happy we were that he was finally here. AJ was born on 4/21/2014 at 10:10 p.m. He weighed six pounds seven ounces and measured nineteen and a half inches.

Adjusting to Being a New Parent

We spent the next two days in the hospital. The nurses were amazing. They knew our situation and set Brandon, Alex, and me in a room next to Scarlett. It was a great two days, when we could finally spend some quality time with Scarlett and her family. In addition to spending quality time with my sister and Scarlett's family, I also learned a lot from the nurses, who provided us little crash courses in swaddling, diaper-changing, and feeding. When we finally left the hospital, I was a diaper changing pro! While I always thought of babies as ultra-fragile, it was reassuring to realize they aren't as fragile as I'd thought.

In hindsight, the drive up to Oregon was a great decision. We couldn't imagine taking our little guy on a plane. Thankfully, our drive home was uneventful and actually a lot of fun. It was nice to ease into parenting with my sister and my partner by my side. The four of us made the drive back to Utah, and my sister helped me transition to being a new parent.

While I have helped to raise our four girls, going through this journey with Brandon from the very beginning was, while not surprising, a completely new and exciting experience.

I get asked a lot what surprises me most about being a new father. Honestly, it's the change in my mindset about life in general and the appreciation I now have for life, even during the conception process. Seeing your own son being created and grown from an embryo, and seeing his development during the pregnancy and during his infancy and now into his toddler phase, has made me appreciate how much of a miracle life is. Even though Alex is only eighteen months old, I can't imagine life without this little guy in our lives. He fills our life with love, laughter, and amazing moments that we will cherish forever.

PART TWO

Anatomy of a Birth Story

~~~~~~~

CHAPTER EIGHT

Master Narratives

I
N OUR CULTURE OF STORYTELLING, certain types of stories get embedded into our consciousness and become master narratives.

Take the American Dream. We all have a blueprint of this story in our minds: go to college, land a good job, make good money, get married, have children, do better than our parents did. If unexamined, this master narrative becomes an expectation we have for our own stories, our own lives. And to some degree, we compare our own lives to this cultural script.

The master narrative can be both supportive and destructive. We can use the master narrative to glean a sense of the arc of a shared experience, and it can help us form and shape our own narratives.

In the case of birth, for example, the master narrative can give us a vague sense of what birth may be like for us or how to make sense of our birth.

Yet the problem with master narratives is that they can provide unrealistic expectations for what our stories should look like— and worse, they can stigmatize, marginalize, or silence anyone whose lived experience doesn't match up.

Our culture has a master narrative about birth that often excludes the actual voices and experiences of the women doing the birthing.

When we dare to tell the truth about our own experiences, we have more influence on the master narrative of birth than we might imagine.

When enough of us dare to speak and write our experiences, which perhaps do not conform to the master narrative, that narrative begins to change.

Rather than me spelling out the master narrative of birth, it will be more useful for you to examine what *you* believe to be the master narrative of birth, and in your specific subculture, given your family, your community, the time in which you are birthing, and the other factors that have influenced the dominant view of birth in your world. The master narrative isn't the narrative you have *created* about birth; it is the one you have been *given* about birth. You are the fish and the master birth story narrative is your water.

I encourage you to examine the waters in which you swim (or did swim at the time of your birth experience).

What do you feel is/was the dominant view about:

- **Pregnancy:** How are you supposed to feel/think/act? What information is available to you? Are you working outside the home? What is your relationship to your partner? How is self-care conceived? What is your prenatal care like?

- **Labor:** What is considered normal? Who are you with? Where are you? What is the role of medicine in your labor? What are you supposed to do/think/feel/believe?

- **Birth:** Where should you birth and by what means? Who is there? How are you supposed to behave? What are you supposed to do/think/feel/believe? What is most important?

• **Birth support:** What is the role and presence or absence of your partner? Doula? Midwife? Medical staff? Family members? Friends?

• **Breastfeeding and its alternatives:** What are you supposed to do? What happens if you can't do that?

• **Immediate postpartum:** Who cares for you and for how long? Where are you? What is considered important? What feels unvalued or invisible? What are you supposed to do/think/feel/believe?

• **The first days and months (and even years) after birth:** How are you supposed to talk/not talk about your experience? How are you supposed to mother? Father? What should your other roles look like? What is supposed to be your relationship to work outside the home?

To access what you conceive of as the master narrative of birth, you may consider what you've seen in the dominant media about birth (in TV and magazines), the attitudes and messages offered by medical professionals and other birth professionals about birth—and your birth in particular—and the attitudes and messages offered by your family and friends (though the latter may or may not represent the master narrative). It may also help to think of what the master narrative of birth was in your mother's or grandmother's generations compared to the master narrative at the time of your birth. You may also examine what is considered normal where you live compared to the birth narrative of a different part of the world or culture.

Here is what one woman wrote about how she saw the master narrative of birth:

> *You're supposed to want a natural birth, but there is a lot of fear about the risks. Some people praise the medicalized in-*

terventions offered in a hospital setting, so there is pressure to comply with how birth is managed medically. A doctor I saw in my first trimester basically told me an out-of-hospital birth was an irresponsible and dangerous choice. But there is also this huge pressure to have an all-natural, intervention-free birth. There is definitely an expectation that my husband should play a certain role in our birth, like be super-involved and know what is happening. On TV, birth is portrayed as this terribly painful and brief experience, with dramatic breathing and savior coaches. There are a lot of expectations about birth in our culture. Everyone has an opinion, and they are usually not afraid to tell you. I'm worried I'll feel like a failure if my birth doesn't go a certain way or if I am not able to breastfeed easily. I feel like no matter what, as long as I have a happy baby, I'm supposed to be happy.

JOURNAL ACTIVITY

Your turn. In your journal, write about what you consider to be the master narrative of birth (perhaps by answering any or all of the questions above). Next, write about how you feel this narrative influenced your expectations and lived experience of birth. Instead of measuring yourself against it, measure it up to the truth of your experience (making yours the default). What do you think is bogus about the master narrative? In what ways did it shape what you expected about birth? What do you wish was the master narrative of birth in your culture?

As you consider the master narrative with respect to your lived experience, remember that your story is legitimate and valuable regardless of how it measures up to the dominant cultural story we have about birth. Don't let your story's non-conformity hold you back from sharing, accepting, or feeling validation for your own experience. (That validation may just have to begin inside of you.)

We need the unique voices each of us bring about birth (especially the truths that exist outside the master story) in order to create a more inclusive, nourishing, positive narrative of birth in our culture. We need more than an ideal, one-size-fits-all birth story. We need all voices at the table.

We need your truth, the TRUTH, in our collective birth story.

In Alex's story below she references how the dominant narrative shaped her expectations of birth, and how she was surprised that things were not as she expected. This helps reveal how the master narrative colored one woman's experience of birth. Her story also demonstrates how the story layers, discussed in Chapter 10, can be woven together.

ALEX'S STORY

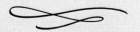

After four consecutive meals of Scalini Restaurant's famous "labor-inducing eggplant parmesan," I started to accept that none of the old wives' tales were going to send me into labor. Pregnancy felt like an eternity, and I was more than ready to meet little Tucker Brett as soon as we could medically call him "full term." Patience has never been a great strength of mine.

My entire pregnancy, I had convinced myself that he would be born two weeks early. I made this educated guess simply based on the fact that my mom had told me that I was two weeks early and I wanted him to be here as soon as possible. Thirty-eight weeks came and went, and so did thirty-nine. One disappointing and *painful* cervical check after the next, I started to feel like my body was never going to prepare itself for his arrival.

As my due date neared, my husband and I started taking vigorous walks on the beach. I began opting for the steep stairwell when walking my dogs in the neighborhood and, to be honest, that I was volunteering to walk them at all was unlike me. I was going to walk this baby right out if eggplant parm wouldn't do the trick.

On my due date, I went in for my check-up and finally learned that I was a whole two centimeters dilated and fifty percent effaced. Two centimeters had never seemed so huge to me and I left feeling like I had accomplished great things with all my speed-walking. At this point, I had been having mild contractions for days. I never found them to be painful, just a tightening of my stomach to let me know something must be happening.

After the appointment, naturally, we decided to have another go at a beach walk, and I hopped into the car to head to one of my husband's favorite surf spots. He decided he would go for a run this time, and I was going to walk briskly, so we chose a meeting spot and headed in opposite directions.

It was a beautiful day and I remember being thankful for that time alone with little Tucker in my tummy and the waves crashing on my feet. I remember ogling the multimillion-dollar houses all the way down the beach and wondering if they were going to fall into the sea one day. I remember wanting to save a rock from the beach *just* in case today was the day that Tucker would come; I would have a special rock to remember it by. I grabbed a couple, looked them over fastidiously, and chose one that still looked pretty even after it was dry. I remember the rock looked like it had freckles. I have freckles so I thought that maybe little Tucker would have them too. We left the beach shortly thereafter—windows down, a warm sunny day in February, with a shiny black rock with freckles in my hand.

I remember asking my husband if we could get sushi that night. After all, you never know when it could be our last opportunity to go out to dinner! I remember he went grudgingly because he never feels like sushi fills him up. There was a cute baby at the table next to us. I stared at him, longing for my baby to be here soon. My husband stared at his tiny meal, longing for a bigger one. The waitresses were fawning over us with excitement once they learned that it was my due date. We saved the receipt from dinner, *just in case*. I could keep it with the freckled rock.

Once we got home, my contractions started to pick up. For some reason, my doctor had told me that it's not "real labor" until I'm toppled over in pain, which consequently left my husband questioning whether what I was describing was the real thing. He decided he would go to bed and "get some rest," while I stayed up excitedly downloading contraction-timing apps. Sure enough, as the night went on, my contractions became more painful and closer together. I decided around 2:00 a.m. that it was time to wake him up and go. I freshened up a bit, realizing that it might be the last time I would have that opportunity for a few days, and I gathered my already neatly packed belongings to head to the hospital. I put my hair in two French braids thinking that would be the most comfortable for being in a hospital bed—and it wouldn't hurt to have it look decent for pictures, either. I woke my husband and assured him that this was the *REAL THING*.

The drive to the hospital was surreal. The world was quiet, dark, and still at that hour, but we were both about to go through perhaps the most life-changing moment of our lives. The pain got worse on the car ride, and I remember gripping the "oh shit" handles in the front seat like my life depended on it. The funny thing about contractions, I learned, is that you feel perfectly fine in between them. Those minutes in between are quite deceptive, and you feel like you can carry on a normal conversation. This conversation lasts only until the next one hits, when you realize it was a ridiculous idea in the first place.

The commute to our hospital is about a forty-minute drive, and to make matters worse, one of the major freeways just happened to be closed that night for construction. I remember thinking, *Is this a sitcom or real life?!* After we navigated our way through the detour and found our way back en route to our destination, I vividly remember the sight of the exit sign coming and thinking, *Hallelujah, pain relief is near.* I should have prefaced this entire story by saying I never had any intention of having a natural birth and have no moral qualms whatsoever about epidurals.

My excitement was short-lived when I realized that not everyone at this birthing hospital was acting with the same urgency that I thought they should. I was just another new mom coming in to have a baby who was told to wait. We were sent up to Triage, or what I lovingly began to refer to as "the place where they determine if you are worthy of being upgraded to Labor and Delivery." Being in Triage is all somewhat of a blur of pain and impatience. My contractions were very close together at this point and terribly painful, at least by my standards. I remember switching positions on the bed every thirty seconds in an attempt to alleviate the pain. Nothing worked. Finally, they came and did a cervical check only for me to learn that I was STILL only three centimeters. How was that possible? *All this pain and NO GAIN*, I thought.

I never thought I'd be grateful to be Group B Strep-positive, but that seemed ultimately to be my ticket into Labor and Delivery that night. Despite having made little progress in dilation, their eagerness to get me hooked up to the antibiotics swayed the decision to admit me.

A nurse finally came to get my husband and me to take us to our Labor and Delivery room. When I realized they expected me to walk, I remember thinking, *What, no wheelchair?* That's not how I had seen it in the movies! We made our way to the elevator and up to the floor where I would spend the next eighteen hours.

The room was gorgeous. Much prettier and bigger than I remembered from our hospital tour several months prior. I remember seeing the warming bed where MY BABY would go when he would arrive any hour now. It was all so surreal and exciting. I remember going to the bathroom, where they asked me to leave a urine sample, and coming back out having forgotten to do just that. I guess my mommy brain was already setting in.

Shortly after arriving in our luxury L&D room, I was set up in my bed with my IV antibiotics. Next order of business was getting something for the pain! I knew it was too early to get an epidural, so I ultimately ended up getting a fentanyl drip. This made all the difference, though its relief was short-lived. My husband took before-and-after pictures of me lying in the bed, and in the "post-pain-meds" shot, I have this ridiculous cheesy grin on my face and am giving him the peace sign. He threatens to use it for blackmail to this day.

Labor was not at all like I envisioned or how I had seen in movies. It was actually a relatively quiet and restful (albeit uncomfortable) day. I was impressed by the level of personalized care the nurses gave me. I knew my nurse had other patients, but it felt like she was just there for me. Whatever I needed—from ice chips to ginger ale, to water or a pillow—my nurse would produce it within minutes. Was this a spa or a hospital? Because I sure wouldn't mind coming back for some R&R!

After a while, the IV pain meds just weren't cutting it anymore. They were wearing off more quickly, and the pain was getting stronger when they did. I don't remember how many centimeters I was at that point, but I know the progression was still slow. We decided it was time to get the epidural, and the anesthesiologist was promptly summoned to my hotel, I mean hospital, room.

The epidural was another aspect of the birthing process that I had seen more than once in TV and movies. I envisioned an image of a woman hunched over, gripping her husband's hands while they plunged a needle the size of a pencil into her back. I was not looking forward to this. It didn't help that my medical-supply-selling husband had already shown me an epidural needle on several occasions, proudly exclaiming, "And *this* is what they will put in your spine." Gulp.

Cut to the epidural going in, and I experienced only a minor pinch of pain. Either I was a total champ, or I was still benefiting from the previous pain meds. The epidural provided a more constant relief from the painful contractions. I didn't have to feel it wearing off every twenty minutes, and when I did, I had a handy little button that would give me another dose of the good stuff.

Throughout my labor from the beginning, there were signs that baby wasn't responding well to the contractions. His heart rate would drop during the bad ones, and the nurses were constantly having me flip from side to side and putting on and taking off my oxygen mask. It was concerning, but he always bounced back quickly once I did roll over. The challenge was staying in a position that he liked and I could tolerate.

The day went on and on. I napped here and there, and so did my husband. When I was uncomfortable, I sniffed the lavender oils I had brought, and they seemed to lull me back into a borderline peaceful state. One of the silly things I remember enjoying about this experience after nine months of being pregnant was being hooked up to a catheter. This may be the first time anyone has ever used the words *enjoying* and *catheter* in the same sentence, but for a woman who was getting up to go to the bathroom an average of five or six times per night, this was a welcome vacation from having to pee!

After hours and hours of waiting for my labor to progress and watching the baby's heart rate drop periodically with the contractions, they decided to administer Pitocin to speed up the process. I should mention that I went into the hospital not attached to any particular birth plan, knowing that I trusted my doctors and nurses to help me make good decisions for the baby and me. This attitude served me well, as I ended up having to go with the flow a lot in those eighteen hours.

Pitocin was not as awful as I had heard it was, presumably because I had already had an epidural. I still was not progressing to the point that they would have expected me to, though, and the baby's heart rate continued to drop with each strong contraction. The decision was made to put in an internal fetal monitor to see just what baby was doing in there. Enter my first negative experience at the hospital.

Shortly after this decision was made, my nurse returned to the room with the internal monitor and two sidekick nurses. I was told that the sidekick nurses were learning how to put in internal monitors (WHAT?) and asked if it would be okay if they had a go at it. Perhaps I was a little too "go with the flow" at this point, because I said, "Sure." I mean, they were nurses, and it couldn't be that hard. After several attempts to get the monitor in and connected to baby's head, the sidekick nurses decided that they just couldn't get it right. Later, when Tucker was born, we would find three little scratches on the top of his head from all their failed attempts. I was not pleased.

Eventually a doctor who meant business came into the room. She definitely had a bit of a doctor superiority complex, but I didn't mind so much after having Tweedle Dee and Tweedle Dum probing around "in there" aimlessly for the previous ten minutes. She got that monitor in within seconds, and we were back in business.

Around 7:00 that evening I *finally* progressed to ten centimeters. I remember it being much less climactic than I had envisioned. My husband was out getting a cheeseburger, and the doctor and one nurse just calmly told me it was time to push. NOW?! My husband had literally been sitting with me for seventeen hours at that point, and he just went to get some food, and NOW it's time to push? I needed to buy some time, and that is exactly what I did.

My husband did eventually return from his journey to the cafeteria, and unbeknownst to him we had gone from a state of waiting to a state of GO TIME while he was away. He choked down his food as the doctors prepared me to start pushing. This was also much less climactic than I had envisioned. The doctor and nurse then got me into the position to push and explained how to do it. I hadn't even pushed a full three times when the doctor stated with authority that it was time for a C-section. Similar to when I had contractions, the baby was not responding well to the pushing and was showing signs of being distressed now.

Everything happened so fast from that point on. One minute there were four people in the room, including myself and my husband, and the next, probably ten. The anesthesiologist was back and doing something to my epidural to numb me entirely from the waist down, and the nurses were dressing Brett in scrubs for the operating room. In an attempt to calm me down, the nurses kept smiling and saying things like, "Now he is just misbehaving in there, isn't he!?", but their inauthenticity and attempts to soften the urgency just scared me more.

Before I knew it, I was flying out the door of my beautiful hotel, I mean hospital, room and being whisked towards the OR. Brett was being shuttled off in another direction, and I was on my own at this point. The fear began to rise. My body was shaking uncontrollably, and the tears started to come. I hate, I repeat *hate*, crying in front of other people, so I did my best to keep a straight face as they wheeled me into the operating room and began to prep me for surgery. Finally, Brett was allowed back in the room and was by my side. I reached out and grabbed his hand for comfort. Except it wasn't his hand, it was the anesthesiologist's hand. Everyone chuckled. I did not.

It was a matter of minutes, some pressure and pulling on the other side of the curtain, and our Tucker was here. I will never forget seeing him come around the side of the curtain for the first time as they placed him on the warming table to clean him up and trim the umbilical cord. Brett got to stand with him while they did this, and I waited patiently for them to bring him to me. My tears of fear were now tears of joy. I couldn't hold him because of the position I was in, but they brought him close to my face so I could kiss him and breathe him in. He was the most perfect baby I had ever seen.

It wasn't long before he and Brett were taken away for measurements and weight, and I was left to be stitched back up. For some, this time away from baby may have been bothersome, but I was on such a high of pure joy that I wasn't even bothered that I had to stay for the completion of major surgery. I made conversation with the staff, I was thanking people left and right, and we made placenta jokes. It was the most radiating and utter happiness I had ever felt in my life lying on that operating table, knowing my baby was just a room away.

Once I was transferred to recovery, my sweet boy was brought to me, and I was able to hold him for the first time. I remember he was wide awake and stared into my eyes as if to say, *Hey, it's you!* I remember at one point he started to crawl towards my breast, presumably to nurse, and I panicked and told my husband to get the nurse because I had no idea what to do. Breastfeeding is one of those things you really can't prepare for until you are in the moment.

After about an hour and a half in recovery, we were taken to the room where we would spend the next three days together as our family of three. It was a tiny room filled with a tremendous amount of love. Over the next several days, the three of us would get to know one another amidst the flurry of visiting family and friends, and nurses and doctors. I remember being a little sad when we were leaving to go home, thinking that we would never have those days again. Three days where we all lived in a tiny room, and our only job was to care for one another. At least we had plenty of leftover eggplant parm at home to ease the transition.

CHAPTER NINE

Birth Story Narrative Arc

*D*ESPITE HAVING JUST OFFERED A CRITIQUE of the master narrative, I am about to give you a tool, a frame, which is the master narrative of all master narratives. Bear with me; I'll explain. This tool is *the* narrative storytelling arc. This storytelling arc was developed ages ago and has been adopted as the governing form of story in oral and written tales, plays, music composition, and even human activity and ritual across time and space. Most of us have a deep internal sense of this narrative arc.

In its simplest terms, the narrative arc of a story is such: story begins, story has a middle, and story ends. For some of us, this may be structure enough to work with as we write our stories. Throughout the ages, humans around the world have sought to develop and refine this most basic of storytelling structures. For example, the Japanese concept of Jo-ha-kyū provides a framework that governs everything from drama and literature to tea ceremonies and martial arts. Our western narrative arc was born in ancient Rome, when drama critic and poet Quintus Horatius Flaccus (Horace, to his pals) advocated a five-part structure to stories. Throughout the centuries to follow, great minds tinkered with this structure, adding and subtracting parts until it seemed to settle again on five parts, when 19th-century German novelist Gustav Freytag created the dramatic structure many of us learn in school.

Before I go on to describe this narrative arc and how you might apply it to your storytelling, let me say I see this going one of two ways for you. One, this tool helps you create a map or plan for writing your birth story. It gives structure to your experience and helps you create cohesion and meaning from it. It is just the form you need to move forward in writing. Yay! Two, you learn the rules to gain the freedom to break the rules. You intentionally make great departures from this form because that is precisely what your creative expression needs to make truth from the raw material of your lived experience. Yay! Either way, may this serve as an invitation to make your story your own.

What follows is an exploration of the five-part classic narrative arc and how it may relate to your birth story, based on what I have seen in the hundreds of stories I have read.

The Opening

Exposition

The exposition of a story introduces important background, such as information about the setting (time and place), events that occur prior to the main plot, and the characters' backstories. This element of a story can be conveyed through dialogue, flashbacks, characters' thoughts, background details, or the narrator simply telling the story.

In birth stories, many people skip this part and go straight into part two (when labor begins). This is all fine and good, but when birth storytellers take the time to include this exposition, it is often rich and vital to the rest of the story. Many birth stories that include exposition introduce a critical framework, a lens through which the writer sees her story and through which she invites her reader to see her story. For this reason, the exposition phase can be so crucial and reveal so much of how we are shaping the current version of our birth tale.

What we say in this first part of our story will profoundly influence what we have to say in the rest of the story. For example, if we begin by writing about how our mother always spoke positively about her experience giving birth, we might more clearly see how we drew on her perspective as a source of strength during a more challenging moment, how it led to certain choices during our birth, or the degree to which her experience compared or contrasted to our own. If we begin by writing about a previous pregnancy loss, that experience can be a thread throughout our story. We can come to see and to process how this past loss influenced and shaped our current birth story. By changing our frame, we may learn something about ourselves we would have otherwise never discovered. Consider how Billy opens his story with meeting the mother of his child (on page 47), Jason's background details about his relationship and family (page 77); Aubrey's summary of her previous births (page 28); and Lauren's opening with a previous birth loss (page 113).

Throughout the many birth stories I have read, common frameworks or themes have emerged:

- women's knowledge/perception of their own births (i.e., when they were born and what they were told/not told about their mother's pregnancy and birth)

- the cultural messages they've received from their families (especially mothers) and their cultural spheres of influence (friends, media, education, partners)

- their personal ideology, beliefs, hopes, and expectations about pregnancy, birth, womanhood, and motherhood

- their previous pregnancies, births, or losses

- their experience of this pregnancy, which may include their experience of conception (particularly if it was challenging), their healthcare experience (specifically their relationship to key care providers), their health, their last few days or weeks of pregnancy, and important moments or aspects of their lives while pregnant

- their relationships with key people in their lives, such as partners, parents, friends, family, co-workers, and other children

- other major events in their lives

Those who choose to write about these topics as a way to open their stories offer a peek into the richness and complexity of their lives outside the vacuum of the birth experience itself.

After all, our births do not occur outside the lives we live, so why should our stories?

For those wishing to process and reflect on their stories, and especially those wanting to heal, I strongly encourage the inclusion of a framework or background that feels appropriate and meaningful to you. You can use this frame as the wild card as you write various versions of your story, playing with how this lens affects what you write.

Imagine if Billy had not used the lens of his relationship to Lisa in his story. Consider how different his story might be if he had focused on the perception of teen pregnancy in his school, for example, or had compared his experience of his son's birth to the birth of his daughter fourteen years later.

Over time, the lens through which you view your story can change, which changes the story itself (discussed further on page 147). When I first wrote my story (page 149) just days after birth, for example, my lens was how challenging weeks forty-one and forty-two were for me as I awaited my daughter's arrival. It was so immediate that it heavily influenced my story's expression. I could have also told my story through the lens of having experienced a previous birth loss, or my worry over losing Maia as I bled for the entire first trimester, or my choice to have her out of hospital. Now, three years later, after losing my ability to have another child, the lens may be how this was my one and only birthing experience and how grateful I am to have had this beautiful experience of becoming a mother.

You'll likely find that whatever lens you use reflects your current thinking and feelings about your experience and all that has come before and after the birth of your child. Often the lens we choose indicates to us something important and alive in us that is seeking expression, processing, and perhaps resolution.

JOURNAL ACTIVITY

List some of the lenses through which you view, or could view, your birth experience and write a few words, phrases, or sentences about each. How would these lenses influence how you tell your story? Which ones are you called to explore further?

The Hook

Another technique I have seen writers use to open their birth stories is the hook or the teaser: a line or short paragraph that draws the reader intensely into the story and makes them want to read more. This hook is often foreshadowing the climax of their stories: a time of great struggle, conflict, risk, or other intensity. Brandon does this in his story, featured below.

If this hook is a device you'd like to play with in your opening, home in on the most potent part of your story, perhaps a moment where the fates hung in the balance or a moment when you were truly tested, and offer a glimpse of that—one that inspires curiosity about the consequences or outcome of that moment—before spanning back to a more chronological telling. You may also choose to open with a mysterious or unlikely setting, some interesting details about a character in your story, or even a thematic statement that hints at what deeper meaning you have gleaned about birth, motherhood, or fatherhood.

JOURNAL ACTIVITY

Where does your story begin?

BRANDON'S STORY

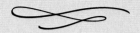

What I remember was the silence.

I remember thinking the silence was strange because of the number of people bustling about. The doctor and a couple of nurses were taking care of my wife Shelli. Four other nurses, maybe more, were calmly but quickly taking care of my newborn son. I stood at the foot of my wife's bed, staring at the stainless steel and ceramic tile walls of the delivery room. I was rattled, but I didn't want Shelli to see I was nervous. Nervous? Hell! I was scared. When a child is born, you don't want to hear silence. You want to hear crying and laughter and cheers and "Congratulations, Dad!"

All I could hear was my heart thumping in my chest and the prayers in my head pleading that he was okay.

Our first pregnancy was just too easy. I understand only a man can say a pregnancy was easy, but as pregnancies go, it was smooth. Excited and nervous as we were, things seemed to go as planned. There was a bathtub, an aerobics ball, a midwife, hippie music, and a delivery room that looked like a hotel suite. Shell did it all without an epidural, and it was pretty much perfect, and our little baby girl was perfect.

So when we found out we were pregnant again, I was convinced we were that couple that has easy pregnancies. Yes, I know there is no such thing. Did I mention I am a man? Seriously, I thought we had this thing licked. The plan was good. We were on schedule to have our daughter potty-trained before our new one arrived. Vacations and sick leaves were all set for the new arrival. With a due date in early March, Shelli would miss being "very pregnant" in the heat of summer. She had the added benefit of celebrating the holidays with a good excuse to eat anything she wanted.

The Saturday before Christmas we were about to leave for some last-minute shopping. Shelli was on the floor with our daughter, and she said something didn't feel right. She didn't act shocked or scared, but I could tell she was concerned. We called the doctor, and fifteen minutes later we were at the hospital. Ten minutes after that Shelli was on bed rest for the foreseeable future. She was in premature labor and needed to be on IV medication. But even then, I wasn't panicked.

Concerned? Absolutely. But I'm a cockeyed optimist and figured all we needed was time, medicine, and a deep breath. Shelli was just pushing herself too hard, and this was God's way of telling her to slow down. *Got it! Message received! Thanks, God. We'll see you in March.*

Not so fast.

After making sure our daughter was squared away at a friend's house, I began calling family to let them know Christmas plans had been altered. I still remember telling Shelli's mother about the premature labor. "Oh, no. It's so early," she said.

The words were so faint that to this day I'm not sure she even knew she said them out loud. That was the first time I got nervous. That is when the questions started flooding my head. *Early? What does that mean for the baby? Would there be birth defects? What kind of defects? Could they be mental or physical? Eyes? Ears? Arms? Heart? Lungs? EVERYTHING!* In that moment, I realized how much I didn't know.

The next few days, while tedious, were also very special. We sat in a hospital room trying to watch TV or talk. There were obviously talks with doctors and ultrasounds and shots. Shelli even had her hair washed by a nurse, and they caught the water in a twenty-gallon trash can: the things you remember. There was also a lot of laughing and hand-holding and hugs and tears.

Most of the time was spent choosing a name. Well, a girl's name at least. As agreed upon before we were married, if the first child was a girl my wife would get to pick the name, and if it was a boy I would get the honor. The other spouse would choose the next child's name, regardless of sex. Each of us had veto powers. Since we chose not to learn the sex of either of our children, it was important to be prepared. I always knew my first son would be named Daniel. But I had never selected a girl's name and, in my defense, I thought I had eleven more weeks to decide.

So we embarked on a quest for a girl's name. There were dozens we liked, but more we hated. Names with "history" got nixed. Former girlfriends' names were out immediately, go figure. We had a whiteboard up so we could visualize the names. It turned into a game. Once we narrowed it down to five sets of names with no clear favorite, we let the nurses vote. If our baby was a girl her name would be Sela Rose. For the record, my wife used veto power on my first choice, Matilda. I still think it was a mistake.

Wednesday morning, we got good news. Shelli got to go to the restroom and take a real bath. She literally cried with excitement. The labor looked like it had stopped, and we had a girl's name. It was the most optimistic we had been in several days.

Then all hell broke loose.

We had a couple of visitors that morning. Shelli started feeling uncomfortable. A little while later, the doctor confirmed that labor had started again. He explained that it might be possible to slow the labor, but it was unlikely we could stop it again. His suggestion was to have this baby and deal with any issues that arose.

Again, my mind started racing with possibilities. We took a deep breath and said okay. For the next couple of hours, Shelli kept progressing through her labor. The doctor and I spent most of time at the foot of her bed talking about the Harry Potter books we had just read. Did I mention the doctor and I were both men?

It was time. Contraction intervals, dilation centimeters, and effacement ratios were all aligned. There was no hippie music, no midwife, no aerobics ball in the corner. There were doctors and nurses wheeling Shelli into what looked like an operating room. There was stainless steel and lights and tile and a small bucket at the end of the bed. There was a team of nurses waiting in the corner. Everyone was in scrubs, and there was a sense of urgency. In short, it was entirely different from our first pregnancy.

At twenty-nine weeks, our baby was obviously not very big. The delivery itself was relatively short. After a couple of pushes, it was welcome to the world.

After a quick look, the nurses whisked him away.

Daniel was here.

The doctor turned his focus to Shelli, and the nurses had Daniel under a heat lamp, doing what they do. I faced the wall trying to catch my breath.

There was the silence.

Why wasn't he screaming? My daughter had screamed immediately. I didn't know much, but I knew he was supposed to scream. Pleas and prayers were still pounding. I stood there for what seemed like ten minutes and heard nothing. It was just so damn quiet.

"Woohoo!" was the first thing I heard. It cut through the air. It wasn't Daniel but a nurse. It was followed by "He's peeing, Dad. Daniel's peeing."

Finally came the faintest cry. A wail or a screech or whatever you want to call it from his tiny little lungs. Then everything came rushing in. I heard him and the nurses and all the other sounds surrounding me. I didn't know everything that was to come, but I knew right then he was crying and peeing, and I've never felt more relief in my life. I wiped my eyes and walked back to Shelli.

Daniel was taken to the NICU (Neonatal Intensive Care Unit) for further assessments. As soon as we were settled, we got word from the nursery that Daniel weighed three pounds, nine ounces: more optimism. That was huge for twenty-nine weeks.

We knew it was going to be a while before we got to see him again. We also knew he had ten fingers and ten toes and a little goat stuffed animal, a gift from the staff. He didn't need a respirator, and that was everything. It would be seven weeks we before we got to take him home. Seven weeks of hospital gowns, NICU beds, hand sanitizers, IVs, and doctor's rounds that made us appreciate both our kids that much more.

The next day was Christmas. Our neighbors broke into our house to wrap the presents Shelli and I had bought each other. We could see Daniel only a few hours a day, and our daughter was at her grandmother's. So we spent that Christmas eating snacks, watching movies, sitting quietly, and feeling grateful for the shower of blessings that was raining down up on us.

I had a beautiful wife, a wonderful two-year-old daughter, and my son Daniel Darrow York. And it was quiet. This quiet wasn't scary, but calming and peaceful like a good quiet should be.

Brandon's hook is powerful. Starting with that scary silence, he beckons us into the intensity of this moment, inviting us to *feel* it, then draws back to provide some background information about his wife's previous pregnancy.

We want to read more; we want to know if his son is going to be okay. He draws us in with this silence and uses it as a hook, a frame, through the rest of his story. It feels cohesive and complete as he compares that first silence to the calm and peaceful one at the end.

Rising Action

The second of our five-part narrative arc is the rising action. The rising action is a series of related moments that build toward the point of greatest interest: the climax. In storytelling, these rising action details are the most important, since the entire plot depends on them. The richness of a birth story, like life, lies in the journey, not the destination.

We all know you'll give birth, but how do you get there?

What is it like as you move through the familiar yet unique landscape of labor and birth and make it your own?

One's journey through the labyrinth of labor is typically the rising action of his or her birth story. To be whole, this rising action piece of your story will likely touch on all three levels of story depth described in the next chapter—the external landscape, your internal landscape, and the deeper meaning you create from the two. In other words, this part will touch upon what happened, what you thought and felt about it, and what it meant then and/or means to you now.

Climax

The third of our five-part narrative is the climax, which is the turning point and is described as the moment that changes the protagonist's or main character's (i.e., your) fate. Nothing tops the fate-changing effects of a child entering our world! Thus, the birth itself is often the climax of a birth story. In the general storytelling world, the climax is described at the point where, if things had been going badly for the protagonist, things start to unfold in her favor, often requiring her to draw on her inner strengths. In a birth story, this may mean that labor has been difficult and demanding, and the birth represents the point at which the laboring woman gets relief and experiences the triumph after her monumental effort.

While the birth itself is often the climax of birth stories, this is not always the case. In some birth stories, a complication or situation that happens before or after the birth is the time of greatest intensity and serves as the turning point in the story. This is where the protagonist must draw on his or her inner strength to move through the unexpected. In Brandon's story, the moment that Daniel cried could be considered the climax.

JOURNAL ACTIVITY

What is the most potent moment in your story? What changes at this time? Why is this moment so important?

In writing your own story, don't feel confined to the idea that the actual birth must be the climax or the most important moment. I encourage you to consider, what is the pivotal moment in *your* story?

You might even choose to write only about the climax, either as part of your processing or as *the* version of your story you wish to tell. Nick does that in his story on page 197. He uses a device called *in medias res,* which brings readers right into the middle of the climax, the middle of the action, and leads from there. At the beginning of his story, Nick brings us into the intensity of his waiting–pacing, eager, and nerve-racked—to see his wife before the birth of his third child, and carries through until his baby boy is born.

Sometimes this distillation of the most potent moments of our story can be a powerful exercise in processing our experience.

Falling Action

The fourth of our five-part narrative arc is the falling action. Falling action, comprised of the events after the climax, wraps up the plot and leads to resolution. In most cases, this is the immediate postpartum period, but this of course could look very different depending on one's experience. Consider the "trial of errors" Lance experienced (story on page 74) in the first hours following the birth of his child.

The falling action may contain a moment of final suspense during which the final outcome is in doubt. This could be a moment of complication, or some hiccup (or major bump) in the road following birth. Perhaps the well-being of mom or baby is in question for a time, or the days and weeks following birth involve an internal or external conflict or complication. This may be resolved or unresolved. Notice in Lauren's story below how the NICU trip makes up the falling action of her story.

LAUREN'S STORY

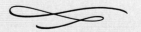

Cecelia's story actually starts a year before she was born. In February 2012, I was elated to see that blue line on the pee stick that meant so much more to me than a simple "positive." We had created life, and I felt so giddy, only to be devastated about six weeks later when my OB told me to prepare myself for a miscarriage. I was heart-broken. I include this detail because, for me, it is a part of the story of how Cecelia was brought into this world.

From day one of that first pregnancy, I kept a journal, chronicling the emotional rollercoaster of life and loss. A few months later, when I learned I was pregnant again, I tried not to get my hopes up, but I couldn't help feeling this overwhelming sense of joy and wonderment at how things must so perfectly align to create life. (I still sit in awe at how babies are such miracles!)

Despite losing my first so early on, I had loved that baby with fervor. That love only grew stronger when I found out I was pregnant for the second time. Cecelia was a strong one right from conception, and she continues to prove that to us at her current age of five months old. The pain of the miscarriage, followed by the hope that came with new life growing inside me, kept me grounded through the following nine months of my life.

My miscarriage experience is part of Cecelia's story, and someday I will share with her the handprints that both she and the one who came before have left on my heart.

That being said, by the time I hit thirty-eight weeks, I was crawling with anticipation, desperately wanting to meet my little girl—to discover what she looked like, learn her personality, and love her to pieces. I have to smile thinking about how our birth doula and Bradley Birth instructor, Nichi, had repeatedly told us to prepare to go to forty-four weeks so that I would not feel that anxiousness that I just described. Ha! I am the kind who plans, organizes, and executes, so when it seemed like baby was going to stay in there all comfy and cozy forever, I tried everything I could think of (within reason) to strongly encourage her way out.

This taught me lesson #1 as a new parent: you are no longer in charge. That little tiny human, yeah, the one who relies on you for everything—s/he's the boss!

After attempting to use acupressure points, vigorous daily walks, squatting, inversions, and the ball, and trying to talk baby out, my due date—Valentine's Day—came and went. Two days later, as I was becoming resigned to the fact that I could be facing two more weeks, my husband Aaron and I decided that a shot at sex couldn't hurt and might actually help. Well, I still contend that this is how Cecelia's *birth*day got rolling. You know those doulas and midwives who tell you what got the baby in there also gets them out? They are right! Within about thirty minutes, I noticed I had lost what I thought was a part of my mucus plug, my forewaters had broken, and I had started mild contractions.

One of the things that I was dying to experience in the labor process were the contractions. It probably sounds silly that I was excited to experience the pain of labor, but for me, experiencing those contractions and the pain to follow was a sort of rite of passage into motherhood that was incredibly significant for my personal growth and transition into a place in my life where I felt more confident and secure with who I was than I had ever felt before.

Of course, now looking back, I know I felt pain, but I can't for the life of me recall the specific sensations. I guess that's why a few days after giving birth I was ready for another one!

From the onset, my contractions seemed to be somewhat consistent, coming every five to eight minutes or so, with the occasional longer period of about ten minutes. Aaron, my loving husband and supportive labor coach from the start, faithfully timed each contraction with his handy-dandy app he had downloaded weeks prior in preparation for this event.

A fly on the wall would have witnessed me sitting on the toilet and yelling to Aaron downstairs, "Start!" and "Stop!" as each contraction passed.

My contractions started around 12:30 p.m. on Saturday, February 16. At some point in the afternoon, Aaron called our midwife, Amy, and Nichi. Amy suggested I go for a walk, have a bath, take a nap, and eat something. So we bundled up and went for a short walk around the pond near our house, stopping every couple of minutes to let a contraction pass, and then continuing, chatting and enjoying each other's company.

After that second walk of the day for me, I took a bath, and Aaron made me some scrambled eggs while we played a board game and watched one of our favorite shows, Friends. I tried to do as I was told to help move things along, but a nap was just not going to happen. I couldn't lie down comfortably. Sitting on the toilet or the balance ball or standing and swaying were the only things that felt comfortable. I didn't know what to make of this, because at the time I thought the timing and the fact that I had to stop what I was doing during a contraction meant something significant. Clearly they weren't that bad when I could take a bath, walk around, and make food without too much of a bother.

At some point, as the contractions got a bit stronger, I realized I needed counter-pressure on my hips. During every contraction from there on out, I had Aaron standing behind me pressing the sides of my hips towards the centerline of my body. It was the only thing I wanted throughout the entire labor process. Aaron was a trooper for never once complaining that his arms hurt or that he had to drop everything he was doing to be at my side the moment a contraction came on.

The way this daddy showed his love and support for me, the mother of his child, was almost as amazing as the work my body did to bring Cecelia into this world.

By 8:00 p.m., Aaron was getting antsy to leave for the birth center, probably nervous that he would get stuck delivering our baby on the kitchen floor, like one birth story we had heard. Around 9:00 p.m., we decided to make the thirty-minute drive to the birth center. We made plans to meet Nichi, her apprentice, Eve, and our birth photographer, Annie, there. The car ride was interesting, to say the least. We made it there without issue, but I remember spending the entire ride sort of bracing myself and grabbing hold of the handle above the door during every contraction, as Aaron was not able to give me the counter-pressure I so desperately wanted in that moment.

When we arrived at the birth center, Amy checked me, but per my birth plan, I did not want to be made aware of how far I was dilated or effaced; I had not been checked during my prenatal appointments up until that point. Later, after the birth, I found out that I was only at three centimeters when I got there around 10:00 p.m.! I'm glad now that I hadn't known then. Keeping this in mind, Amy asked me to start walking the stairs, two at a time, to help me open up.

I started making my rounds, up the stairs, around the yoga studio on the second level, back down the stairs, and repeat. When a contraction wave hit, Aaron faithfully squeezed my hips as hard as he could while Nichi and Eve dropped to all fours to provide a tabletop support for me to lean over. At some point, I said I only wanted Aaron to be squeezing my hips, because he offered the strongest vice; I'm not sure if I actually said this out loud. In my memory I screamed it, while I'm sure in reality, if I did say it, it was probably pretty quiet.

I moved into the shower, and just as I did, another wave came rumbling through me; immediately Aaron dropped to all fours, fully clothed, to support me on the wet floor of the shower. That night, I think Aaron would have gone to the ends of the earth for me if I'd asked him to; he was such a strong and silent rock for me during this journey (and still continues to be).

There was a definite point in the labor experience when I recall allowing myself to let go and give in to the pain. When I started to release control, I hadn't even realized that I had been holding on so tight for all the hours that had come before.

It was in the shower where I think baby and I did most of the work. During every contraction, I would move into a deep squat and allow the physical sensations to take over. I know I kept asking to get in the birthing tub for some relief, and I could tell Amy and Nichi were trying to hold me off. I also remember turning to Aaron multiple times and telling him that I just wanted to be done, that I couldn't do it anymore. I also kept thinking to myself, "If I were just in a hospital, I could get an epidural!" For the record, I am so glad I was not in a hospital and that pain medications were not available to me!

I spent the whole time in the shower with my eyes closed, focused within, unaware of most of what was happening around me. I spent the rest of the labor experience with my eyes mostly closed, almost in a trance-like state, focusing only on the present, moment to moment. I had no idea what time it was or how many hours had passed. Once I moved from the shower to the tub, I got some relief and was even able to fall asleep in between contractions. Most of this time is pretty foggy for me. I have bits and pieces of memories of loud vocalization, feeling as though my arms were shaking (I don't know if they actually were), and being reminded by Nichi to relax my face and bring my voice down low. All the while, Aaron and Nichi took turns sitting behind me on the edge of the tub, supporting me and switching out the cold washcloths that Eve dutifully continued to rewet with ice-cold water all night long.

If you're ever wondering what a doula can do for you (um, besides the invaluable job of providing undying support and encouragement), remember that they are great at feeding you and keeping you hydrated! Eve held the water bottle up to my lips, fed me bits of dried fruit and other concoctions that she and Nichi had packed in their bags, and she even put my hair in a ponytail and moistened my lips with Vaseline on demand.

I think Amy assumed it would be a while before this baby was coming out, so sometime when I was in the shower, she and my other midwife, Monica, decided to take a snooze. I think my animalistic noises surprised them, because they hadn't expected me to be in transition so soon. By the time Amy checked me in the tub, I was starting to feel the urge to push. Amy gently told me there was a small lip left on my cervix (I was at nine centimeters), so I couldn't push yet. So here I was, following Amy's instructions to "puh-puh-puh" (that's the best way I can describe the sound she told me to make with my mouth to avoid bearing down during every contraction). To help things along, Amy held her hand against the cervical lip during each contraction to assist in full dilation.

Then it was time to push. I pushed in the tub, I pushed on the bed on all fours (that's when I started throwing up), and I pushed on the birthing stool. Then Amy recommended that she put in an IV to give me a sugar boost because I had been throwing up and was losing steam. I remember even from when I started pushing in the tub that I could feel the hair on my baby's soft head when I reached down after pushing. I recall checking over and over after every surge of pushing to see if she had moved any farther down, and I started to get frustrated that nothing much was changing. While on the birthing stool, I was given a mirror so I could really see Cecelia's head making its way out. I could tell that Amy kept moving me from one position to another because things were sort of stalling. I wouldn't say that I ever lost confidence in my ability to bring this baby into the world on my own, but I started to struggle with catching my breath in between contractions and pushing. Luckily, I had a team of people surrounding me on the birth stool, encouraging me, telling me how strong I was, that Cece was right there, and reminding me to slow my breathing. I clearly recall feeling that "ring of fire" we had heard Nichi talk about during the Bradley classes, and then sweet release as the rest of her body came sliding out of me.

In the end, I had moved to the bed, lying on my back (who would have thought this was what would do it?!) and I pushed my beautiful girl right out into Aaron's waiting hands. Cecelia Marie was born after sixteen hours of labor on Sunday, February 17, 2013 at 4:30 a.m. at seven pounds, six ounces and twenty-one inches. I took her in my arms, and I couldn't see anything else around me but my beautiful baby and my wonderful husband. The discomfort of Amy massaging my uterus and the shot of Pitocin in my leg to stop the bleeding was far overshadowed by the intense attachment and feeling as if I already knew this little person so well.

Despite the fact that Cece was so alert, gazing at me with her big, wondering eyes, she never screamed out. She was given a few puffs of oxygen, and we held an oxygen mask on her face for a while, but we never heard even a whimper. Perhaps she was more intrigued by this whole new world of hers than shocked, so a scream wasn't necessary. She didn't immediately latch on, either. She really just seemed to be taking it all in and savoring the process with no urgency to cry or feed. That's really who she is to this day—my silent observer, just taking it all in (my friend calls her an "old soul").

Because of this so-called "respiratory distress," which wasn't really distress at all since she was breathing on her own and her heartbeat was good, the non-emergency team from Children's Hospital was called, and they asked to take her back to the hospital just to make sure everything was all right. I was in baby-love land, so I handed her over after cuddling with her for an hour. Aaron and Nichi went with Cecelia to the NICU while I stayed at the birth center for a couple hours to get cleaned up and eat something. No stitches were needed, so I showered and ate a yummy ham-and-cheese croissant that Eve ran out and picked up for me as soon as Bread & Chocolate opened at 7:00 a.m. I later realized how much I had needed that refreshment in order to face what was coming next.

When I walked into the NICU room, the nurse was putting in a feeding tube to administer formula to Cece. I lost it. This was not in the birth plan! I wanted to breastfeed and bond with my baby, and when I told the nurse this, she snapped at me that my baby needed this, and it couldn't wait (but props to Aaron for advocating on our behalf and refusing to let the nurse give a bottle). This nurse made it sound like a matter of life and death, which it obviously wasn't, since babies are born with a full tummy. When Cecelia had arrived at the hospital, they couldn't find anything wrong with her. The only thing that came up was low blood sugar, and guess why? Because she hadn't had time to nurse after birth yet! But in my fragility as a new mama, I didn't have the energy to fight any more than that. So that was it. My baby was just given formula for her first feeding.

I had a good cry, then picked myself up and told the nurse that Cecelia would not be receiving any more formula; I was determined to make breastfeeding a success.

From there on out, Cece successfully breastfed, and guess what, her sugars were higher with the breast milk than with the formula, wouldn't you know it! We stayed in the NICU for the next twenty-four hours for "observation," and they still couldn't give us any good reason why Cece needed to stay, other than to watch her sugars. This baby was not sick, clearly. We stayed about twenty hours longer than we really should have. If there was one thing I wish I had done differently in this whole experience, it would have been to follow my gut and walk myself and my baby right out of that hospital, because being poked and prodded for the next twenty-four hours for no good reason, in my book, was not an enjoyable first day of life for any of us.

This was lesson #2 as a new parent: trust your gut. You are the parent, and you know your child best— you can give your child what they need more than any doctor or nurse can. Little did we know as we left Children's Hospital the next day, it would not be Cecelia's last visit. Two weeks later we were back in the hospital, as Cece was diagnosed with Hirschsprung's Disease (a condition affecting the large intestine that causes problems passing stool) and needed surgery. She had a follow-up surgery at four months old. But, as I already mentioned, my little bug is a strong and resilient one, and I can just about guarantee that she will be a stubborn and driven adult, doing things in her own way in her own time. I will always be one proud mama.

If you have made it this far through my story, congratulations. You are either a mama-to-be who is biding your time before you meet your little joy, or you are a mama who has a baby nice enough to allow you a few minutes to yourself for renewal and decompression. Either way, I appreciate you sticking it out with me. One of the ways I renew my spirit as a mama is by reading amazing and inspiring birth stories.

For me, it gives me a sense of community with all you other mamas who care to inform and educate yourself about the world, your fellow women, and yourself—your preferences, your beliefs, and your value as a bearer of life. Pregnancy, birth, and parenting is a journey, and albeit hard, it's rewarding as heck. Now, five months later, I am still loving mommyhood. Having Cecelia has given me a purpose and a drive I never knew I was missing before she came into our lives.

I have never felt as confident or secure in who I am until I became a mama. Something inside me just clicked and told me, "You have it all; be content and satisfied." And I was. Still am.

Resolution or Revelation

Also called denouement (which means *to untie* in French), this fifth and final part of our arc, called the resolution or revelation, includes the events from the end of the falling action to the actual ending of the story. During this part, conflicts and complexities are often resolved, creating a new normal or new reality for the protagonist. This is also the time of catharsis, or the release of tension and anxiety, in the protagonist, in the reader, or both. In the birth story, the resolution may be considered the "new normal" of life after the birth of your child.

In birth stories, this final part of the narrative arc may include anything from the time following birth. This may be where a writer reflects on and derives meaning from their birth experience, as many of the stories in this book do. Some writers will here include what wisdom and importance they draw from their stories. This is the most natural place for most people to dig into story bones territory, which we discuss in Chapter 10. Some may offer advice to other women (or men) about birth or parenthood as Vanessa does on page 217.

When Resolution Has Not Come

For those of us with birth trauma, this resolution can be the most difficult aspect of storytelling, because there is a pressure to wrap everything in a pretty bow and show how you are better now than you were before, how everything is okay. But if things don't feel better, and things aren't actually resolved in your life, they cannot be resolved in your story. While the act of writing itself can lead us closer to a resolution, to closure, there are times when we need to leave our story bittersweet. If this rings true for you, let me suggest that you remove the pressure to include this ending for as long as you need to. Instead of wrapping things up in this perfect pretty package, talk about the current complexities and complications. What is alive for you right now? Talk about the here and now exactly as they are true for you, no matter what that looks like.

As you write about your experience through time, you may find that you make some steps, however small, toward resolving conflicts and tensions in your heart and in your story. Or perhaps they remain, and you establish a different relationship to them. Consider the raw, soulful ending to Kelsey's story on page 141. She acknowledges the heartbreak and the darkness while also revealing the light and the healing.

Part of being a woman, a mother, a human, is embracing the paradox, the co-dwelling of the dark and the light together in the same moment.

JOURNAL ACTIVITY

Where are you in the dance between the dark and the light, both present in the intensity of bringing new life into the world?

CHAPTER TEN

The Birth Story Layers

IN ADDITION TO HAVING A NARRATIVE ARC, our stories also span various landscapes and levels of expression. Here, we explore the three layers of a birth story: the surface skin, the mid-layer of story muscle, and the deepest layer, the story bones. For another presentation of this information, please also check out the chart in Appendix B.

Top Layer: Our Story Skin

The skin of our bodies is what is most easily seen of us and what we reveal to the world; it covers and protects our deeper structures. The skin of our birth stories is also the outermost layer, what we most often show of our experiences and what serves to protect the deeper aspects of our truth.

This story skin is where "what happened" takes place—it is the keeper of the facts, the timing, the setting, the chronology, the what, where, when, and with whom.

Our story skin, comprised of these facts, is what any observer might see of our story. Like skin, it blankets the story in a surface layer of continuity—it could even be seen as holding the story together, offering a container for all the deeper structures. Our story skin is often what we feel most comfortable showing the world.

The story skin speaks in nouns and verbs; it loves quantity over quality; it favors the concrete and the physical.

The story skin registers the external landscape of our experience—what we can see, touch, hear, feel, and taste.

In the context of storytelling, the story skin correlates with the setting, context, and action of our story. At the skin level, we are the actors, enacting roles and displaying traits by performing behaviors in the presence of others.

We all begin our stories at the skin. We need this place as our starting landscape, as the first thing we encounter as we explore the body of our story. The facts provide the physical landmarks we can use to guide ourselves deeper into the terrain of our experiences and come back out again. We need to know how it happened—when labor started, what the day was like, how long our contractions were, how long we pushed, who was there and what they did, what time baby was born, her weight and length.

The story skin is also the acceptable social script from which we are expected to read. When someone asks, "What was your birth like?" we are expected to answer from our story skin—our answer must reflect the surface-level facts, not the heart or soul of our profound experience. Just the facts, ma'am. See women's comments on pages 26 and 27 for examples of this expectation.

Without reflection (and courage) many of us remain at our story skin. Like our actual skin, the story skin covers and protects what lies beneath. Given the deeply vulnerable nature of our birth stories, most of us deem it safest to stay on the surface. We can use our story skin to hide behind, to keep people out, to keep ourselves disconnected from the deeper layers of our experience. This may be appropriate self-protection—just as our physical skin keeps the bad bacteria out, sometimes sharing only our story skin with another protects us from the non-supportive response we risk in revealing what lies beneath.

While the story skin can protect us socially, we must remember that it requires a degree of permeability to let in the goodness—like how our skin absorbs vitamin D from the sun. Opening past our story skin can offer nourishment, such as fulfilling our deep need to feel heard and seen by others as we reveal the tender, vulnerable aspects of our experience.

"I spent a lot of years trying to outrun or outsmart vulnerability. . . my inability to lean into the discomfort of vulnerability limited the fullness of those important experiences that are wrought with uncertainty: love, belonging, trust, joy, and creativity, to name a few," writes vulnerability research pioneer Brené Brown.[1] The possibility of fulfilling these fundamental desires—to be loved, to belong, to experience joy—lies beneath the skin of our stories.

> In our data-driven world, it is easy to mistake the chronology of events for our actual birth story. This is not your birth story.

It is the scene in which your *experience* unfolded.
Let's dive deeper.

Middle Layer: Our Story Muscles

Sometimes when we share birth stories, we want to tell and we want to know, what happened medically, interventions, outcome... but we often overlook the importance of the more subtle sub-story of various relationships before, during, and after the birth.
PAM ENGLAND

Going a layer deeper, we move from the external landscape of our experience—the facts—to the internal landscape of our experience:

our thoughts, feelings, needs, relations, and the quality of our experience. Our story muscles reveal how we feel and what we think about what happens to us. This layer of our story is like the muscles and connective tissues of the body in that they serve as the prime movers of the body. They generate and coordinate action and the effects of such action, they protect what lies even deeper, and they store and release energy.

The female body is made of approximately forty percent muscle (for men, the percentage is even higher). So are our birth stories. Our hearts and wombs are some of the strongest and hardest-working muscles in the body. At this layer, we begin to get to the heart of our stories, to the womb of our stories. Our story muscles—our thoughts, feelings and how we relate to the external—needs voice in our narratives so we don't atrophy in our growth. Without these underlying dynamic movers and coordinators, our skin is lackluster and lifeless.

The story muscles speak in adjectives; they love quality and nuance.

The story muscles point toward the heart of our story: the emotional, mental, and relational realms.

In the context of storytelling, this layer correlates with character development and mood. These enrich our story. At this second level, we are the agents of our story, acting upon inner desires, goals, values, and plans.

The story muscles are dynamic and changing. Some of them fall under our control, while others function outside of our intention—just as our thoughts and feelings may arise without our intending them but be essential to our survival.

This layer is woven throughout the body of our story but can look different in different places and in different stories. In one place, the muscle is meaty and robust as a key driver of our action; in another place, the muscle is not as developed or relevant to the action in question. What is meaty and what is lean depends on the writer and her story. For a parent with a full-term, healthy baby, a mention of baby's length and weight in her story may not register heavily in her internal landscape, but for a parent whose child was born early or has trouble nursing, baby's weight is of the utmost importance to her internal landscape.

How this inner landscape looks and how it is captured on paper is deeply personal and highly variable. Some people will feel at home in this layer and find ease in putting words to the inner world. Others may feel awkward or challenged by exploring this unseen but powerful level of experience. It can take courage to get to the heart (muscle) of our stories and bear the truth of this layer. But the benefits of this reflection can be tremendous.

Muscles and connective tissues are anything but static—they are fluid and dynamic; they are changeable. Our thoughts and feelings are also fluid and dynamic. Here we unearth the seeds of our liberation—from victimhood, shame, and limiting belief, should they factor into our internal landscape.

We may not be in charge of our skin layer (the external), but we can wrestle with, claim control over, gain compassion for, and even reinvent our second layer.

As the agents in our story, we get to create its shape and learn from what it reveals to us. We can discover how we felt and what we thought in the course of our actual experience. And then later, as often as necessary, we can rewrite our relationship to the skin of our stories, choosing how we feel now, choosing to cultivate new thoughts and feelings, make new meanings and connections, and draw new insights. Here we can make our story our own.

Many of the stories in this book, such as Hope's below, offer great examples of the story muscles at work. Hope demonstrates how key the story muscles are to the expression of our birth experiences. She couples nearly every element of the story skin with the story muscles, her inner landscape of thoughts and feelings.

HOPE'S STORY

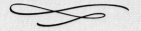

When we started the adoption process, I had to let go of the idea that we would get to witness our baby come into this world. I knew there were plenty of adoptive families who didn't even meet their children until after they had been born. Of course, this was challenging, since as a doula and an expectant mother, I desperately wanted to be hanging around when the big moment happened. I felt like I was going to explode when C invited not only me to be at the birth, but Zach, too. This was going to be the best birth I had ever attended, no matter the birth outcomes. Because it would be the day that my daughter was born.

The week of November 2, C asked us if we were feeling ready. Zach said that we were mostly ready and that we would be packing our bags for the hospital that week. Of course, I rolled my eyes at this. My doula-self thought, *we probably have plenty of time; there is no rush to pack for the hospital. We could probably pack the moment we get the call and still have plenty of time to drive about four hours to meet C and our little girl.* I am not sure why I thought this, since I normally like to be prepared, and Zach is the procrastinator. In any case, I was completely overwhelmed with all that still had to be done for the benefit that weekend, not to mention working on several grant applications that were calling my name now that we finally had our home study done. Somehow the day before the benefit happened, Zach convinced me to pack my bag and a bag for baby girl. (At this point we still had no name for her.)

Our friends and family arrived for the benefit from every corner of the state, and some of them from out of state. We laughed, we cried, we ate, we drank, we danced. We partied hard. After we cleaned up and got home, Zach crashed, and I was pumping. I had been working on inducing lactation to nurse this baby girl and at this point was pumping ten to twelve times a day to prepare my body for the arrival of a newborn baby. While I pumped and reveled in all the fun Instagram pics from the night, I got a text from C.

"You wanna see something gross?" My doula-self got butterflies instantly. I knew something was up. "YES!" Then ensued a photo signifying that labor (too much information for you regular folk) *could* start happening soon. I smiled and got very excited and nervous. I elbowed Zach, "Sounds like things could happen any time now. Good thing you made us start packing some." Zach rolled over and went back into a deep sleep, without ever recalling a thing I said. C and I texted for a long time that night. We were both giddy. The baby could be arriving soon.

The next day I packed more stuff and made a list of the essentials we needed to remember. Bottles, pump stuff, the car seat (a gift from Zach's co-worker, which we still needed to pick up), a gift for C, and all the essentials for staying in a hotel until paperwork was signed and we could cross state lines to bring our baby home. I went to the mall to choose an outfit to bring our baby girl home in—something small just in case she did come soon. I was standing in Carters when my phone rang. It was C.

My heart skipped a beat.

"Don't freak out."

"Okay?"

"Everything is okay right now, but I am having some signs that something might be going on with the baby. I am going to go in and get checked, but I want you to know that based on my research, they may want to induce me today. Tell Zach not to worry. I will keep you updated about what the hospital says."

Of course, I worried. I knew Zach would worry, too. When I called him, we agreed that we should just drive to Austin and stay at my parents'. That way we would be close in case an emergency did happen. We didn't want to risk missing the birth. We prayed that our baby would be okay and that C would be healthy and okay, too.

That afternoon, Zach wrapped everything up at work so that he would be ready to go on leave. I finished my shopping and errands. My best friend Lizzie came over—she would be coming with us to be my doula and to photograph and film the birth (C is amazing and allowed her to do that!) so that we could share the whole story with our girl one day. She helped me calm down and then humored my obsessive-compulsive nature and helped me nest. We did a quick deep-clean of our whole apartment so that it would be baby-ready. We drove to pick up the car seat and met Zach at work.

We got to Austin late that night and went to bed exhausted. We waited the whole next day. Still no news. At the end of the day, C got test results back. She and the baby were completely healthy. She felt bad, though. She had wanted it to happen for us and knew we were so excited to meet the baby. She was feeling ready to be done with the aches and pains of pregnancy. I assured her we were completely fine; we were so thankful she and the baby were healthy, and we were happy to wait as long as it took. This was sort of a white lie, since Zach was really sad that he had to wait longer to meet our little girl. He was also sad that he had to go back to work.

We took the next day back at home getting our house more officially ready for a baby, doing a few "must-get-done" projects. I was so thankful to have a little more time. We had just breathed a sigh of relief that things were coming together.

We had only been home for a day when C called.

Zach and I were crazy nesting at home. We used our last moments sans baby to hurry up and buy a king-sized bed (since we would most likely be needing the extra space to share when we would bring a fussy baby into bed with us). Then we went to Target to pick up the last baby essentials and sheets for our new bed. We ran into Zach's cousin, who had been through the adoption process herself not that long ago, and she gave us some kind and encouraging words. I appreciated that so much; it helped to calm my nerves.

We were putting on our new, just-in-time-for-winter flannel sheets when my phone rang. It was C.

"Don't freak out."

I was beginning to get used to this phrase, so I wasn't too anxious at first.

"Okay," I said with a huge grin on my face.

She proceeded to tell me that she was bringing her kids somewhere, and on the way there her water broke. Of course, I knew that this was the real deal. There was no going back now. If her water had indeed broken, there would be only a number of hours before our baby would be born. And I believed C because she had done this before. She knew what she was talking about.

Commence me starting to freak out (internally, of course).

"Okay. Okay. Uh-huh." I could barely listen to the rest of what she had to tell me. Our baby was really, really coming. And hopefully we wouldn't miss it! We still had to drive four hours.

She was on her way to the hospital to confirm that her water had broken, and without hesitation we re-packed the car—this time we were much more ready. We felt like we had everything we needed, and our house was pretty much in order.

I will never forget that day. It was gorgeously sunny outside, with crisp fall air and a bright, clear blue sky. I looked around as we were leaving our apartment and saw that it was as organized and clean as it ever would be. Our freezer was completely stocked with meals I had spent weeks preparing. The nursery was ready—even though we knew she wouldn't be sleeping in there for a while. I had butterflies. The next time we walked through the front doors of this place, it would be with a baby.

I grabbed all the milk I had pumped and saved for the last few weeks from our freezer. (I'd proudly saved about twenty ounces already!) We locked our front door, slammed the trunk of our Subaru, and hopped in for the ride of our lives.

We could hardly contain our excitement. We updated our closest friends and family about what was happening. We prayed together for C and for our baby girl. We narrowed down baby names to two final options and decided we would make the final choice when we saw her face. Then we would know for certain.

We took a selfie, both giddy as schoolchildren, and posted it on social media with no explanation—this is as close as we could come to sharing our excitement publicly since we were not allowed to share anything on social media about the details of our match.

Surprisingly, the car ride flew by. I was so thankful for that.

We pulled into the hospital parking lot. Lizzie (if you recall, my best friend, doula for me, and birth photographer/videographer) was already there, waiting to capture our arrival on film. I was so relieved to see her there. I knew she would help me stay calm.

We got into the room, and not a lot was happening. C was calm and happy and did not seem to be contracting often. It was really nice to see her—to see that she was doing okay—and it was a relief that we made it in time to see this baby be born. I was glad that C was not in agony, but I was also a little worried that there were still no contractions happening. My doula-self had looked into the cesarean rates of the hospital that she would be birthing at, and I was alarmed to find they were 46%. I had to let go of that.

C's boyfriend (not the baby's biological father) was there to support her, and I was so thankful for that. I wanted her to have someone there with her just for her. He was so loving and supportive of every need she had. She deserved that. They decided to go walk the halls along with Zach and Lizzie, to see if they could help things pick up. Meanwhile, I pumped.

When they got back, C put in her headphones to listen to her birth hypnosis tracks that she had been practicing. I could not be happier that she wanted to use hypnosis for this birth—both for her sake and for the baby's. I wanted this to be as relaxing and without fear as possible for her.

I offered to give her some massage and make the mood more relaxed in the room. I got out some candles and essential oils. I can't even describe to you what this experience of serving the mother of this baby was like for me. It was such an honor for me to be present with her and to attempt to comfort her while she was about to endure a huge sacrifice that would change our family forever.

The hospital staff came in and discussed starting Pitocin, as they were not satisfied with how things were progressing at this point. C agreed to that. She still tried relaxing through each contraction, but they were much more intense now, and it was becoming increasingly difficult to do so.

After a few hours of this, she asked them to turn the Pitocin off. She was tired and she wanted to rest. I was so happy for her that she was strong enough to advocate for what she really needed most at the time, and that was to sleep. The next morning, after we'd gotten a few restless hours of sleep, they talked about turning the Pitocin back on. C decided that she wanted an epidural. She was worried about how I would feel about this. Of course, I assured her, this was *her* birth experience, and she should absolutely do whatever she felt was necessary. I could not imagine being in her shoes—it was completely different than if I were in labor myself. I truly wanted her to have whatever she wanted to be the most comfortable. She deserved at least that.

They got everything going to place the epidural, and they also started the Pitocin back up. I checked in with Zach, who was by himself in a little waiting room, playing his ukulele and trying to self-soothe his anxiety, which was welling up with each passing minute. He was dying for this baby to get here and to get here safely. He had felt this way since we found out about this baby girl, but it was especially evident in these moments leading up to her birth. He could not rest until she was safely in his arms. We talked, cried, hugged each other.

It was starting to get long. I had been through this at many births before, but Zach had not, and it was wearing on him. I told Lizzie to have Jake (Zach's best friend) call him and give him some encouragement. Jake did, but Zach was still pretty down. Lizzie and I went to get some breakfast. I needed a little food and refreshment to be re-energized. Who knew how much longer this could go? Or potentially, since her water had now been broken for a while, at any moment they might tell us they were going to take her in for a cesarean.

Lizzie and I sat down at a table in the hospital cafeteria. My tray was piled high. I was starving. Just as I was about to take my second bite, and we were deliberating about how everything was going, C's boyfriend came rushing into the cafeteria.

"You guys should probably head back now. She says that she's feeling like she needs to push."

My jaw dropped.

"What?"

"Yeah, she says you should hurry," he said matter-of-factly. We brought our food with us to the room that we were keeping all our stuff in—a little waiting room with a door that we could close so it was just the three of us. We got Zach and rushed into C's room. I could tell by the look on her face that it was going to happen right then. I asked her if she had updated her doctor about that. She told me that she had. He was chatting it up with a nurse in the hallway. Zach went out to make sure he knew that C wasn't messing around.

It seemed like only seconds passed, and there was a huge team of people in the room with us—labor and delivery nurses, a baby nurse and doctor, and C's doctor. Her doctor put on scrub covers and handed me a glove box as I double-checked with him to make sure that I could still help catch the baby. I was so excited to do this part. Around this time, I told Zach that I would pass the baby; he would be the first to really hold her. I felt that was only fair since I thought I was really getting the better end of the bargain by getting to catch her. I told Zach that he should unbutton his shirt so that he could do skin-to-skin with her right away. There was a look of terror in his eyes.

"It's okay," I told him. "All these people are here just to make sure that everything is okay with the baby and with C."

In just a couple good pushes, we were already seeing our daughter's head. Zach tried to look away out of respect for C, but once the top of the baby's head was visible, he couldn't look away. I could see the awe on his face as the weight of the reality of his daughter finally emerging into this world was sinking in. One of my favorite parts was witnessing my husband—this man that I have loved so much for so long—finally becoming a father.

I had my hands ready to catch her. She was so little. The doctor had his hands right alongside mine to help guide me. It felt like she was so tiny. It was so strange to me to hold her with gloves on. In retrospect, I almost wish I hadn't worn gloves. I didn't want there to be any barrier between her and me. I wanted her so, so much, and she was finally here. The doctor clamped the cord as I held her in my hands, and then I cut the cord (also something that I was so excited to do). Then I took her back, briefly held her up to my chest because I just couldn't resist, and then handed her over to Zach. She was completely covered in white, creamy vernix and still wet with amniotic fluid, so I wasn't sure if Zach would still really be into snuggling her or not. He didn't seem to mind. He snuggled her close, closed his eyes as he took in all that just happened, and wept. I was smiling so big. It was amazing to see him with this baby. Then she peed on him.

I looked back at C, for the first time wondering how she would really be feeling about everything. She just smiled with approval. I still have no idea how she did that. She was a pillar of strength. My admiration for her only increased. At this point, I was feeling happy and excited that this baby was here, but I was still mostly concerned about Zach's experience and how C was doing. When Zach asked if I wanted to hold her, of course I said yes right away. Without a thought, I unbuttoned my shirt so that I could do skin to skin with her too. It did not faze me for a second that there were a million strangers in the room. I needed to get this baby on my skin ASAP. She fit so compactly right in the center of my chest. She *was* little! I sat down with her, snuggling her even closer and drinking her in.

It was in this moment that I finally thought about the feelings I was having, and I realized in my head, *you sweet, sweet baby girl, you have made me a mother. All this waiting. All this heartache. It was not in vain. It was because of you. And you were more than worth the wait.* And I wept uncontrollably. Zach just held me. And when I could finally open my eyes again, there were her big, deep, dark eyes, staring up at me. I had seen many mother-baby pairs experience this before, but to experience it myself was a whole other thing. This baby was connecting with me. I was her mother.

We cried together over this incredible gift that we had dreamed about for so long. Again, I looked at C, thinking that it must have shaken her up to see us both getting so emotional. And still, she was smiling even bigger now, with her iPad out, taking pictures of us with the baby.

After we had spent a little time with our daughter and gotten a little better look at her, we talked quietly between us, making final decisions about what we were going to name her. Without hesitation, I knew what her name should be. She was so elegant and beautiful, with her arms reaching out right after she was born. Zach agreed that it was a good fit.

Estelle.

And her middle name would be Peace—she was so quiet and peaceful, and a virtue name was appropriate since both of her mothers had virtue names. Estelle Peace Lien. C insisted that she have our last name on the birth certificate right away. It fit her so perfectly. We were so, so in love with her from the moment we saw her.

This was really just the beginning.

Deepest Layer: Our Story Bones

At our deepest layer, we find our story bones. Our bones provide the solid frame that holds our bodies, our stories, our lives, together—they provide structure and form. Just as our body's bones are moved by the muscles, the story bones are driven by the emotional-cognitive-relational internal landscape that forms as we experience our birth, our life. In our body, the bones protect what is most vital—our brains, our hearts, our lungs, our wombs. In our story, the bones also protect and represent what is most vital—our sense of what our stories *mean* and why they *matter* to us.

> Our story bones are where we make meaning from experience—what lessons we have learned, what wisdom we have earned, what enduring truths we have gathered from the depth of our experience.

Clarissa Pinkola Estés asserts that, in archetypal symbology, the bones represent the indestructible force. "They are by their structure hard to burn, nearly impossible to pulverize. In myth and story they represent the indestructible soul-spirit."[2] Our story bones reveal our soul.

In the context of story, this level offers the themes, morals, and messages—the wisdom and the truth found in story (see Appendix A for a list of common themes that emerge from birth stories and please add your own). We were mere actors at the skin level, agents at the muscle level; it is here that we become the authors of our story. As the autobiographers of our stories, we can take stock of life—past, present, and future—to craft a story that tells who we have been, who we are, and who we are becoming as a result of our experience bringing a child into this world.

The story bones reside in a deep place of mystery, wordlessness, symbol, and archetype. They are brought to the light of consciousness as we work to put words to this level of our experience. While it may be challenging or feel approximate at best, working at this level is where we gain integration and deep healing.

If we are in need of healing, the story bones beckon us to deep work—to melt away all the details—the connective tissues, the muscles, the skin—to strip down to the skeleton, the bare bones, the essence of our truth. What in our experience is essential? What is true? And when we've gathered these jewels from the depths, we swim back to the surface, reconstructing our stories, re-weaving the skin, muscles, and connective tissues together once again to make new forms.

As clinical psychologist, Jungian analyst, shaman, and author Carl Greer writes in his book *Change Your Story, Change Your Life*:

> *Your life is more than a series of events that happen over the course of time. It is a story with themes and patterns. How you tell your story is up to you, but if you can tell it honestly and are willing to work with the energies that affect your personal energy field, you can write an entirely new story with new themes and new patterns of events [...] Even though you will not change the facts, you will modify your interpretation of them, and your framing of them. The emotional charge of your wounds will be diminished.*[3]

He notes that through writing your story, you may cultivate new emotional energies, such as pride in having survived difficulties and joy in having created something positive out of suffering.

Seeking ways to make meaning from our experiences is a vital part of our processing birth. When we reflect upon the significance of our stories and the insights we've gleaned, we can reap great rewards of understanding, connection, strength, healing, and more. However, there is a certain flavor of meaning-making that is best left out of our birth story recipe. Harmful lines of inquiry can focus on blame, guilt, and shame. Questions like: *Why did this happen to me? How did I invite this in?* and *What did I do to deserve this?* are not fruitful lines of inquiry that yield much benefit. I've also heard the line of reasoning that *because x didn't go as I'd hoped in birth—I had this complication, needed this kind of support, had this kind of intervention—this means that my body is flawed, or I am flawed.* This kind of meaning-making does not serve us well, nor is our reasoning often true. More often this line of reasoning is the result of painful emotions that have not yet been fully processed and can indicate that further exploration and healing support are warranted. I recommend opening the doors to greater self-compassion, empathy, and healing by completing the Non-Violent Communication writing exercise offered in Appendix F. May I also suggest working with a qualified care professional who is trained in supporting one's journey to uncover and shift core and key operating beliefs (see Resources for recommendations).

When you begin to identify the meaning you've created from your story, ask yourself, "Is this really true?" "Does my experience really support this conclusion?" "Can I find evidence in my story or my life that complicates or contradicts the meaning I've constructed?" Here is one brilliant example of a woman working with the story bones.

KELSEY'S STORY

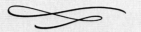

I have given birth three times. Once on an operating table under general anesthesia while my baby was delivered out of me by suction and curettage. Once supine on a hospital bed, pushing for four hours while numb from the waist down, delirious from fifty hours of labor and zero sleep. And once lying on my left side, bearing down in irrepressible convulsion while I roared my baby out with unmedicated ferocity.

My first birth made me a mother. My second birth made me a mommy. My third birth made me a believer.

I cried at each of my births. The first time, the tears were grieving tears. Three days earlier, I had learned at my nineteen-week ultrasound that my baby had died in utero, a full four weeks prior to us finding out. I begged my body to go into labor so I could feel my baby pass through me, the only experiential evidence I would ever have that he was real, alive, mine. The only way I would ever hold him. But my body, like my heart, wouldn't let go. So as the IV dripped into my arm and a kind nurse instructed me to count backward from 100, I wept the tears of bereavement, of a mother telling her child goodbye. I cried because he left.

The second time, the tears were petrified tears. I had only ever known birth as death. I wonder if a lot of mamas who have grieved babies are scared to their very cores as they endeavor to bring another life into being, a formidably brave task. Though the child in me flailed and kicked as if she were at a U2 concert, I just couldn't believe it, couldn't believe her body would come out of me breathing and screaming and pulsating with life. We rocked in a chair and called her by name, that name that means Life itself. I cried because I was terrified she would leave.

The year after this birth, I sobbed rivers of tears as the very fabric of who I was came undone, and I descended deeper and deeper into perinatal mood disorder. I didn't stop crying until God and Zoloft saved my life. Then I cried as I worked my ass off, arranging and re-arranging the pieces until the quilt of myself made sense once again.

The third time, the tears were different. They were not only the tears of grief and fear. They were the tears of redemption, as well. Tears of worship. Tears of Mama Heart. They came on the ball and in the shower—just me, my husband, and the hot water streaming down and intermingling with the hot water streaming from my eyes.

"I found my tears," I said to our birth priestess (our amazing doula) when she met me in the steam. "They are good tears."

"What are you feeling?" she asked me.

"I feel my babies. I feel my love for them, my overwhelming love for them. It's flooding every fiber of me and giving me courage and strength. I feel my love for Samuel. I feel my love for Geneva. And I feel my love for Miriam. They've come to me here, and I'm holding them. I want to hold them and cherish them and pour every ounce of myself out in love for them. It hurts so good."*

---

*Clearly, I didn't really say any of that. I was birthing! More likely, I uttered some jumbled words and groaned a whole bunch. Had I been in my conscious mind, however, this is what I would have said.

These were the tears of love: for the babies, for motherhood, for a life brought back from the brink. These were the tears of gratitude: this birth, the culmination of two years of healing and transformation, without which this baby's life would have never been possible. And these were the tears of visitation: my babies came to me in that shower, every last one of them. This time, as Sammy came to me from Beyond, I got to hold him again in the only way I can now, when I connect emotionally and feel him in my heart.

He was the vapor that filled the room; he was the tears that streamed down my face. I cried because he came, and it was glorious.

There comes a time in every birth when a woman faces her darkest hour. My first birth, that hour came as a needle pierced my skin, and I agreed to surrender to death. My second birth, that hour came as hours stretched into days, and I pushed and pushed and pushed some more and agreed to surrender to life. My third birth, that hour came as a ring of fire, and I finally agreed to surrender to belief. Belief in life beyond death, belief in life after death, belief that I can embrace both life and death in these lionhearted mama arms of mine. Belief that it is possible for a life to be redeemed and remade, to go through hell and come out transformed for good and for the better. Belief in One who redeems, in Spirit speaking to Gut. Belief that I have been made into a Mother, with a body and a mind and a heart and a soul brave and faithful enough to take off every mask as I make my way to the center of the birth labyrinth and bring this child forth.

He came.

She came.

They surrounded me as I birthed their sister into being.

When they placed Miriam on my chest, my entire being came together as the reconstructed quilt that was her receiving blanket. And I wept. On that quilt, there is a Sammy square, an Eva square, a Miri square. Each one stitched with heartbreak and fear. Each one held together also by belief and vulnerability and valor and love.

I cried because they came and because I *be*came whole.

JOURNAL ACTIVITY

What meaning does your birth story hold for you? What new perspective have you gained as a result of this birth experience? About yourself? About others? About birth? About motherhood/fatherhood? What has remained forever altered in you following this birth? What connections can you draw between your birth and your life? What essential truths have you drawn from your birth experience about life?

Weaving These Layers into Narrative

The layers of our narrative refuse to live in neatly stacked boxes. We can't say, *here is the page about what happened, here is the page about how I felt and what I thought, and here is the page about what it all means to me.* In reality, these layers like to be woven together, sometimes with great complexity, as we write our stories. It's bound to feel a little messy.

My best advice is to embrace the messiness, the complexity. Keep these ideas about your story's layers in the back of your mind as you write, but don't let them trip you up. Play with the inclusion of all three layers of your experience as you write; and allow them their natural expression.

The intention of exploring the three layers of story here is to give you permission to venture into all layers of your story, as you desire. Kelsey does this so beautifully. The story skin is revealed in the concrete imagery of that steaming shower, the visual of the kind nurse instructing her to count backward from 100, the timing of her labor progression. She touches the story muscles, the heart of her story—her heart—in the emotions she expresses: her grief and bereavement; her fear and terror; her downward spiral into depression; her redemption, worship, and unconditional, overwhelming love for her babies; her courage, strength, and tenacity; her gratitude. Her story muscles also reveal her inner landscape in the imagined dialogue she has with her doula. She works with the story bones, the soul of her story—*her* soul—in the meaning she makes from her experiences. She is able to articulate and name the kinds of tears she sheds and why; she speaks to the universal core-shaking fear that mothers who've lost children so often experience; she reveals the connection to her children, which knows not the boundaries of time and space; she explores the ways in which we face our darkest hour as women in labor; she reaffirms her faith in One who redeems; and how our births are squares on the quilt of our souls.

CHAPTER ELEVEN

Birth Stories through Time

IME CHANGES OUR STORIES. It's inevitable. What is important to us today may not be tomorrow. What we saw in one way today we will see in a different light tomorrow. What colors the expression of our experience is in a state of constant change.

In many ways, our story processing through time is a journey through the layers just described above, but it is not a linear or clean process. We often find ourselves at varying depths of each layer simultaneously.

We begin without a story at all. During birth, we simply experience it all without any narrative yet attached. Here we may say we are deep in bones territory where no mind-made story resides. Then, as time stretches away from the delivery, we may begin to craft our surface story, pulling together the details and the facts about what happened. We may also dip into the middle layer with powerful emotions about our births and the people around us. We may begin to form ideas and beliefs about our births, birth itself, ourselves, and others.

This is the first pass through the layers. It may be a whirlwind in those early hours and days, which quickly disappears in the cataclysmic adjustment to life with a newborn. Or it may continue to unfold. It may be part conscious and part unconscious. Many of us stop processing our stories, at least on the conscious levels, never venturing beyond our sterile social stories, our birth "elevator speech," the surface tale. Yet there is gold beyond that first mountain.

How much one processes and digests their experience through time depends on the container they are offered or create for themselves, and the value placed on this introspective processing, both in their immediate social environments and within themselves. If we have this container that allows us to make our processing conscious, as through writing, we witness the changing and deepening nature of our stories through time.

As time passes, everything we experience in relationship to ourselves, our children, our partners, and the rest of the world begins to filter into and influence our remembering of birth. Deeper meanings, associations, and perspectives continue to take shape as we place this transformative experience into the context of our lives. Time is a fundamental factor in accessing the rich bone-level insights and meaning making our births offer. Consider the experience of our story contributors who wrote decades after their births. Time was such a significant factor in the dramatic discoveries and healing that Billy (page 47), Betsy (page 15), and Kelsey (page 141) gained by writing, gifts that would likely not yet have been available soon after birth.

So what does this consideration of time's effect on our storytelling mean for us? It's simply important to recognize that time changes our stories, and writing through time can make conscious our ever-changing relationship to our births.

Below I offer just two versions of my own birth story: the first, a detailed narrative written in the first weeks after I gave birth; the second, a poem written more than three years after I gave birth. Notice how different each of these stories is—how the first narrative includes all three layers of a story, but it orbits around the story skin. Notice how the poem's axis is squarely in the bones, with the muscles and skin as secondary and tertiary elements. I know that I could write my story ten different ways today. I know that my story will look completely different in twenty years, in ways I can't even begin to imagine.

Wherever you are, honor it. At all points in time, your story is valid and valuable. There is no expiration date on the expression of our stories, and no time in which they are fully complete, even if we finish writing them.

JAIME'S STORY

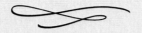

I'm Late

Like many first-time moms, I was fairly convinced my baby would greet the world sometime between thirty-seven and forty weeks and not a day later. For some reason, I had it in my head that February 14, our due date, was the absolute last day she might arrive. This despite knowing first-time mamas often deliver beyond their due dates.

Week thirty-seven came and went as I racked my brain for additional nesting activities—I'd finished my semester teaching at the university weeks earlier, and there wasn't another room to paint, rearrange, or clean in the whole house. At this time, my intuition shifted, too. Though I was uncomfortably large (with a rockin' case of pubic symphysis pain) and baby—we called her Sprout—was sometimes uncomfortably active, I had a new feeling she was quite content where she was. I was unsure she'd ever want to leave her comfortable womb life. Weeks thirty-eight and thirty-nine came and went. So did our due date.

Like a slow-motion film, the days crept by. No baby. Every day felt like Groundhog Day, the same day as the day before . . . again and again. At first I struggled; I was done with this godforsaken Minnesota winter. I was done waiting. I was ready to hold my baby. I was ready to welcome this new chapter of my life. It was crazy-making to spend every moment of every day prepared for labor and this radical life change to happen at any moment—like knowing an earthquake is going to hit, but not knowing when.

I spent a few days working myself into an anxious mess—I wept through an entire lunch date, *in public*, with my hubby. I'd hit a low that wasn't helping anyone, and I resolved to forge a new perspective. So I surrendered. I simply decided to let it all go—the worry, the desire for control, the expectations, and the detrimental internal dialog. I stopped telling myself "today is the day," I stopped expecting labor at any moment, I stopped trying to *will* labor to begin, I stopped pretending I was in charge. I just gave my best to surrender and *trust* in the mystery that is birth.

At about day ten post-due, we had to start facing the reality that if she didn't come in the next couple of days, we wouldn't be able to birth naturally at the birth center. Though this troubled me deeply, I tried to keep a vice grip on my new chosen outlook. We had until Thursday, February 28 to see if we could get this labor started naturally or we'd be looking at a hospital birth with medical interventions.

Inducing Labor

As of the Friday before, my cervix was showing no sign that labor was coming anytime soon. We spent the weekend taking various natural measures to coax baby into the world (sex, evening primrose oil, walks, and acupuncture treatment). No labor.

By Monday morning, my cervix hadn't changed, so we began the natural induction process. For twenty-four hours, I wore a special catheter with two lime-sized bulbs of water pressing on either side of my cervix to coax it to soften and efface (open). The midwives and nurse said that if I opened to five centimeters it would fall out. It didn't. It felt like I actually had the proverbial stick up my butt . . . and my mood matched this reality.

The next morning, day twelve, I was dilated to only one or two centimeters, but my cervix had changed some. They removed the catheter and explained the herbal induction regiment I would begin. This involved taking four ounces of castor oil. The castor oil is meant to irritate the digestive system and so irritate the uterus, ideally prompting the latter into contractions. I would also be taking some homeopathic medications and an herbal tincture, alternating the two every fifteen minutes for four hours.

I was excited and nervous, knowing that labor could be just around the corner. I was advised to take the castor oil with a juice that I wouldn't mind never drinking again. I chose grape juice, since the only grape juice I like is called wine. This combo was like taking a huge swig of motor oil and chasing it with Robitussin. Yet I guzzled down the whole concoction like it was a tequila shot and I was back in college.

It could have been worse.

It got worse.

The effect of castor oil is much like the worst food poisoning you've ever had. Within twenty to thirty minutes or so, I met with something akin to Montezuma's Revenge and spent much of the afternoon getting better acquainted with my bathroom. Quite the humbling and eventful prelude to labor.

Early Labor

But it did the trick. After kicking off the induction process at about 1:00 p.m., early labor contractions began coming every five minutes by about 2:30 or 3:00 p.m. Billy and I spent the afternoon in our guest bedroom watching movies. Well, he was in the guest room, and I was mostly in the bathroom. Labor continued through the afternoon. At about 6:00 or 7:00, we went downstairs to cook pasta carbonara for dinner. I made much of the dinner, stopping every few minutes to brace myself through contractions on the cold, gray-speckled granite countertop of our newly remodeled kitchen.

After dinner, we returned to our little labor cocoon upstairs. I spoke with our midwife, who suggested that I take another dose of castor oil (the opposite of what I was hoping to hear!) but in kindness, she cut my dose in half. By 10:00 p.m., contractions had slowed a bit with some coming closer to seven minutes apart, and I worried labor was waning. But I kept my spirits up. Billy and I decided to try to rest a little. It's amazing that one can actually be in labor *and* sleep: thank you, birth god(esse)s.

Active Labor

By midnight, labor had shifted from early labor contractions to more intense and frequent active labor contractions. They were coming every one to five minutes; some lasted a minute, some a little less. They were much more intense than the earlier contractions and required my focused breathing and vocalization to ride each wave.

Billy, half asleep, offered the verbal support I needed to stay confident and in the moment with each new rush. Like a narcoleptic running a 100-meter dash, I managed to get through the intense physical exertion of a contraction, pass out for a few moments, and be jolted back into wakefulness with the next wave. This lasted only a brief time until I was just up, laboring hard, for the next six hours or so. I stayed perfectly present for each contraction and prevented mind chatter from adding any suffering to the physical pain. I was just experiencing and witnessing this awesome primal process. It was really something.

As the morning sun crept in through the windows of our 100-plus-year-old Victorian home, Billy called our doula, Greta, and they decided this would be a good time for her to join us at the house. Until this point, I'd been laboring solely in the side-lying fetal position with my fist on my forehead, which felt good and safe, but I wasn't sure if it was sufficiently aiding my labor progress. I really didn't want to move, which was surprising since I thought I'd be more active through labor.

When Greta arrived, she suggested we try a few other positions. We went into our bedroom, and I got on the big birth/exercise ball. I didn't like being upright one single bit. The pressure added by gravity was great, and the contractions were more difficult to get through. My mind began to resist, but I tried to trust that this was helping labor progress. Since it was morning, we decided the shower might be a good change of positions, though Greta warned that it could bring on harder contractions. It was hard to stand through contractions, so we brought the ball into the shower. The shower felt great, but labor was really intense so the experience was short.

Afterward, Greta suggested I sit on the toilet and labor there for a while, as it was a good position to keep labor rocking. *Oh, hell no.* I did *not* like this! It was the discomfort of the ball times ten, and I felt too exposed and a little scared.

My mind, which had been largely off-duty on a beach in Mexico until this moment, frantically searched for a way out of this experience. Something. Anything. I tried to negotiate with Greta and Billy—if I could just rest on the bed for a few minutes, I'd promise to return to this godforsaken position if we thought my labor was slowing down.

It worked.

Ah, back to the bed, my safe place. Labor only continued to intensify, and I was able to remain in my little cocoon, wrapped in towels and blankets, howling like a warrior woman, with Billy and Greta watching over me.

At some point, maybe around 8:00 a.m., Billy spoke with our midwife. Because of Billy's calm demeanor in the face of nearly any event, he might have under-expressed the state of my laboring. However, once she heard me in the background she likely gained a better idea of our progress.

Nevertheless, she suggested I try to eat something, and we would touch base again. Greta so kindly spoon-fed me bites of oatmeal between contractions.

I remember keeping my eyes closed, totally disinterested in food, feeling utterly exhausted and increasingly nauseated. In retrospect, I realize I was moving into transition.

Oneness

While feeding me, Greta intuitively asked, "Are you experiencing any strong thoughts or feelings you need to express in order to move forward in labor?" I considered. I could feel my dad's presence very strongly in that moment (he is in spirit), and I tried to communicate an ineffable experience.

I commented, "I know this is going to sound crazy, but I don't just *feel* my dad *around* me, in some weird sense, I feel like I *am* my dad." This sense of oneness with him makes perfect sense to me—not only were my dad and I really close, but I felt I was experiencing the same utter surrender and need for support in birth that he experienced in his death. I understood him exquisitely in that moment.

In the early days with Maia, I also experienced this same sense of oneness with her—like I understood her from the inside and that we were the same person in some way (which I suppose we'd been for quite some time!). Of course, these oneness experiences all unfolded during the process of my bringing forth a separate being from my single body. So, in a way it makes sense. But it goes deeper. Because birth calls us to the threshold between two worlds, we may get a rare glimpse into the Mystery and an *experience* of Truth, in this case that we truly are all one (which is often just a pretty concept in my mind, but here, I *felt* it).

Transition

Anyhow, labor started to ramp up once again, and it felt like my contractions didn't end—they just went from a ten down to a seven and then back up again. I was deep in a place within, tapping my inner reserves for all the strength and energy I could muster. As things got really hazy (and loud!), I experienced something new: pushing. At least two of my contractions on our guest bed went from "regular" squeezing contractions to all-out involuntary pushing.

"I'm pushing, you guys!"

I was astonished and for a moment thought surely I would birth this baby right there on the bed. I reached down to see if I could feel her head. She felt so close.

It was really time for us to go. But that was the very last thing I wanted to do. The idea of actually getting up and going somewhere seemed ridiculous, if not completely impossible. "Please just call the midwives and ask them to come over," I begged. They had to come to us; there was just no way I could move. Despite my certain belief that I was immobile, I had such full trust in Greta and Billy that I complied when they insisted we go to the birth center. They swore that I could do this. I had to do this.

During pregnancy, the transition phase of labor made me nervous—I'd heard it was one of the most challenging times in labor, those moments when you were most likely to feel defeated, if not certain you were going to die. And here I was looking at the prospect of actually getting in the car and traveling to a new place during this phase of labor. Birth brings you right into your fears, forces you to look them dead in the eye, and offers you a chance to move through them. When I knew that I needed to go (and go now!), I rallied and did what I needed to do. I decided that after a contraction subsided a little, I needed to run downstairs and out to the car. I was completely paralyzed during contractions, so this was the only way it would work.

Greta and Billy somehow dressed me, and I was ready to make a dash. I barely made it down our creaky old staircase, before a contraction forced me to collapse onto the hardwood floor for a couple minutes or more. After it slowed down, I jolted up and ran through the backyard's bright morning sunlight, hoping to at least make it to the car before another one started. Just barely. I jumped in my Toyota Highlander and slammed the seat all the way back just as another double overhead transition wave came crashing all around me. This one lasted, no exaggeration, the entire five-to-seven-minute ride to the birth center. It just never let up. I didn't think, I just howled like mad through the contraction and hoped that the baby didn't pop out onto the floor. Once we arrived at the birth center, I had a moment's break to run to the door, through the reception area, into the birth room and hurl myself onto the bed. I barely made it.

At the Birth Center

We arrived sometime just before 10:00 a.m. Through a hazy half-glance, I saw Jill, our fabulous nurse, prepping to check my cervix. "Jill, you better tell me I'm at a ten," I muttered, birth-drunk. She checked and chuckled, "Oh yeah, you are there, sweetheart." It was time to push (some more!).

I had a few more super-intense contractions on the bed, as people came in and out of the room, preparing for the birth. I was happy to see the familiar faces of Amy, Amanda, and Monica, our midwives, and I felt complete trust and peace in the situation. I was in good hands and right where I needed to be.

Water Birth

They drew a bath and suggested I get in for the pushing part of labor. I was happy for this choice, as I wanted to deliver in water if it was a good option for us. Though it felt a little scary to move, I made my way into the tub and got on all fours. I labored like this for a while as contractions turned to full-force pushing. Everyone was around me, encouraging me and helping me focus my energy during each intense wave. Pushing is no joke; it's like trying to move a mountain. Or a continent. Or a universe. I resolved to give it every ounce of my strength and energy, giving way more than I ever knew I had. I pushed with every single atom in my being.

Like contractions before, I had a good, couple-minute break to gather my strength in between each pushing wave. It was in these pauses that I noticed Billy had put on super-chill meditation music. I appreciated the tranquility it supported (though I also could have gone for some pumped-up rally jams, since I was performing the most epic physical feat E V E R.)

My water broke in this position, and the team told me there was meconium in the water. Meconium is poop that babies release in the womb, which can impede their airways as they take their first breaths. Amanda calmly explained that it was going to be okay; they were going to suction her right away to clear her airways, and then they'd hand her over to me.

I changed positions another two times, once to a reclining position the long way in the tub, with my hands bracing myself up and my legs spread. Then Amanda suggested I get into that same position the short way in the tub, so I could really open my pelvis and bring my legs up. I was in that position for another half a dozen pushes or so, I think, before Maia was born. Those last couple of pushing waves were the ultimate finale to labor—I gave everything I could and tried my hardest to push her out quickly but not too fast. Greta later told me she felt like I had this amazing protective energy surrounding me and that I was in a deep place somewhere slightly removed. Looking back, it feels like one of those dreams where you are hovering above your body, watching things happen to you.

I was able to reach down and feel Maia's head a few minutes before she was born. It was indescribable. I held her, crowning, between a set of pushes, which the midwives said would help my tissues stretch. I remember my strongest motivator at this moment was Billy—I could hear the joy in his voice as he caught the first glimpses of his daughter, and I wanted so badly to give him the experience of seeing her. It was a selfless and pure wish for him. (Okay, maybe I was ready, too.)

Maia Is Born

I pushed her out with the next wave. Maia was born at 11:11 a.m. on Wednesday, February 27, 2013. It was an intense physical experience, but I was in the haze. This haze makes it hard to describe with accuracy what happened next—and so many things seemed to happen all at once.

I remember seeing Amanda holding Maia up by her feet. Maia was crying. I didn't see, but I know they suctioned her. Also, the umbilical cord burst when Maia was born, sending blood all over the place. They clamped it, and before I knew it she was on my chest. I don't know if I have words to describe the feeling of first holding Maia. I mean, how do you describe the ultimate miracle? It was pure joy, and awe, and wonder; I loved her instantly and intensely. It was also a shock—*who are you, and how did you get here?* She was more beautiful than I could imagine. I was meeting someone I'd waited my whole life to love. It was so big.

Little Emergency

But the tub seemed to be getting darker and darker with blood, so they asked me to hand Maia to Dad and get out of the tub. I was still completely in the Birth Fog, so I just followed others' directions without much thought.

But as soon as I got out of the tub, saw blood pouring all around me and the flurry of action on part of the birth team, some distant part of me (which was surely back on that Mexican beach) became a bit concerned.

As they helped me to a birth stool, I recall asking if everything was going to be okay, but the Fog blocked true worry from my mind. I birthed my placenta, but my uterus had a hard time contracting as is necessary to avoid excessive blood loss.

I was bleeding profusely, so I received the full treatment—a couple of injections in my thigh and a gritty pill in my mouth, lots of painful pushing on my belly, buckets being filled with blood and tissue—and after a while, the hemorrhage emergency seemed to subside. (Thanks to the competence and quick action of the birth team. Total rock stars.) This experience scared the bejesus out of poor Billy.

Holding New Life

I was helped to the bed and—after a little more serious pushing on my uterus to ensure the bleeding had ceased—I got to hold Maia again. After that, she was really all I could focus on. I was so exhausted and weak, but I just wanted to hold and discover her. Greta helped us learn how to nurse, and we worked on different holds for a while. Maia was a fantastic and eager nurser from that very first try. I am so grateful for that. Billy and I snuggled in to stare in wonder at our new little love. The things going on around me are a little blurry in my memory. Amanda brought over the placenta and showed it to us. (She later encapsulated it for me.) Amy told me lots of important and helpful information I instantly forgot. Greta offered me a tropical-tasting drink and more water. I ate pizza from Pizza Luce. They gave Maia her first physical exam, and she was healthy as could be (though they heard a heart murmur that would resolve itself in a matter of days). Maia weighed eight pounds exactly and was twenty inches long. She had a good cry from the start.

I soon discovered another cause of my profuse bleeding: I had torn badly through my inner and outer labia and a little on my perineum. Apparently Maia stuck her hand up by her head as she was making her grand entrance. Amanda also told me her head had rotated around as she came out of the birth canal, creating a wider space upon passage. Amy spent at least an hour stitching me up—it took at least forty stitches to get the job done. This birth was beautiful but very physically taxing. In all, we stayed at the birth center about five hours after the birth. We left at about 4:30 in the afternoon and headed home. We had great hopes of sleeping soon, as we were told babies usually sleep six to eight hours at home after the birth. Well, she didn't exactly get this message until the next morning. Eventually, after lots of exhausted activity I cannot really recall, we slept from about 4:00 to 10:00 a.m., the longest stint of sleep we'd have for weeks to come.

But our beautiful baby girl is in the world. We had an amazingly beautiful birth experience and came out stronger than I thought possible. Billy was so proud of me in the coming days; it was the greatest feeling in the world. Maia and I did it. We did it together, surrounded in love and support from some truly remarkable people. It doesn't get any better than that. I am so grateful.

JAIME'S POEM

As the waves grew steady and strong at the water's surface
I duck dived down,
Beneath this seeming tumult,
Into the ocean of my being,
Smooth and calm.
I passed the threshold where "I" became "All"
And touched bottom,
The deepest place,
Where from all beings are born.
I called out for your soul to join me
Inside this singular body and
Your light illuminated me from within.
Now fetched, I squeezed you tight and
Pushed
Pushed
Pushed
My way back to the surface.
As we neared the crashing waves again
My body opened for you
Slippery and slender,
You swam forth courageously.
Hitting the air with unreckoned force,
You gasped,
I sighed.
The physical cord linking our bodies burst —
You were singular for the first time.

You cried heartily and
I felt the awe
Of watching a fish learn to breathe.
Though separate in body, our spirits mingled in the water still
everywhere.
Soon that water turned crimson:
It was time to turn for land.
Here I heaved and hoed, clearing myself of the remnants of an
abandoned home,
No longer meant for shelter.
Your father, the sun, held you brightly
As your mother, the earth, shuddered and shook until settled
once more.
You returned to the earth's embrace where you fed from wise
waters
Meant to sustain you completely for days, months, even years,
to come.
You learned to drink steadily and gain deep nourishment
Like you'd known from the tree at your source.
Every molecule of the new air you breathed
Was bursting with
Love
Wonder
Gratitude.
We drank it in together.
We held you in this bubble of bliss until it became us and
We three launched out into the life we'd charted long ago
To walk hand and hand
Here.
Together.
Different bodies,
A singular heart
Pulsing to the rhythm of Love.

PART THREE

How to Write

CHAPTER TWELVE

Getting Started

STORYTELLING DOESN'T HAVE HARD AND FAST RULES, but guidelines. You may be disappointed, but this section does not include a simple formula and specific instructions that make writing a breeze. If you find the simple formula, let me know; I want to see it! What this section does contain are lots of ideas, support for your writing process, and suggestions for what to think about as you write and revise.

While writing comes easily to some, for many it is a daunting task about which we feel reluctant and unsure. We think there is some right way to do it (that we aren't aware of) or that somehow we won't do a good enough job in the telling. We can't seem to find the time to sit down and write, or we don't think it is worth our time to write down our experience of birth. Or—the most tragic in my opinion—we don't think our story is important enough to tell.

Whether you are eager and optimistic about writing or reluctant, I am here to tell you that writing about your birth experience is absolutely worth your time, that your story and your voice are so important, that you absolutely can write your story in a satisfying way, and I am here to help you. There is no wrong way to tell your story, and you know you're telling it "right" when it feels true in your bones.

I firmly believe that the value of writing down our stories comes not in the product, but in the process.

The power and benefits of writing your
birth story don't come in the shiny finished
envelope tucked away in the baby book,
or the number of likes you get when you
share your story on social media.

You create magic (and healing and meaning and value) in the process of writing, no matter how messy or misspelled.

Setting an Intention

Anytime we bring our conscious awareness to why we have shown up for something—in this case, why we are here to write our story—we gain the power to own and direct our experience. Setting an intention clarifies why what we are doing matters and motivates us toward action. And, practically speaking, our intention shapes what we do in our writing.

There are many reasons a parent may choose to write his or her story. We have talked about many of these possible reasons in Part One, but here we are going to really reflect on your personal reasons for being here, for writing.

Here are just a few reasons for writing I've heard from women and men I have worked with:

- I want to find a sense of peace.
- I want to remember.
- I want to find empathy for my experiences, my choices.
- I want to be in this place of heartbrokenness; I want to feel the feelings of what my/our experiences were.
- I want to write about identity shifts and cultural expectations around pregnancy and birth.
- I want to grieve.
- I want to celebrate.

- I want to influence my community with the experience I had birthing my daughter, to show them an alternative to the "typical" birth story.
- I want to write this for my child to read.
- I want to understand more about what happened.

JOURNAL ACTIVITY

What are your reasons for writing? What is important to you about writing your story down? How do you want to feel while writing and after writing?

Once you gain clarity about why you are here to write, consider what you need to support your intention. Do you need time? Do you need a particular kind of support? Do you need to shift your perspective about writing your story? Do you need to give yourself permission? Do you need to work with a group of women writing their stories? Do you need clarity about something? Do you need a plan?

JOURNAL ACTIVITY

What do you need to support your intentions for writing?

Making a Plan

Clarifying your intentions and needs for support can naturally parlay into creating a plan for your writing. We all vary in how much planning will feel supportive. But I invite you to consider how you envision your writing process unfolding and how you can be success-ful. Creating explicit parameters around why we are writing, what we hope to accomplish, how long we wish to write for and at what frequen-cy, and what form we desire our writing to take—all of these produce a structure that can offer us safety and set us up for success. The most effective structures also incorporate a good degree of freedom, so plan and then release that plan, opening to receive it or something better.

In planning to write your birth story, consider the amount of time you may need to write, how often you can commit to writing, and what times of the week or day are ideal for you. Be realistic. What is a reasonable amount of time you can devote to writing and at what frequency? How long do you think you can/want to write each time you sit? What are the best times of day, days of the week? Give your-self freedom to modify your plan throughout your process, knowing that our stories can take on their own lives, guiding their pace at the periphery of our control. Some people will have the luxury of writing their story in one sitting. This can be a helpful way to feel a sense of cohesion in our storytelling, but it is not often the reality for parents. We may dream of heading to our favorite darling coffee shop and writing for hours, but our reality is writing in ten-minute spurts after baby has nodded off at the boob. We may dream of writing on a weekend retreat, but we only have time to write at sunrise before all the kids start screaming for breakfast.

JOURNAL ACTIVITY

Take some time now in your journal to create a plan for your writing process. It might help to consider your ideal and also what feels most realistic for you in your present life. Don't create this plan as a line on your list of "shoulds" or "to-dos" but as a way to empower yourself to make your intentions a reality.

CHAPTER THIRTEEN

Ways into Your Story

S OME OF US WILL SIMPLY WRITE, no prompts needed. We have a vision of our story in our heads, and it's just a matter of getting it on paper. For others, we need a little push, a little jumpstart out of the gate, and once we're off and running we'll make it to the finish line with ease. Others still enjoy a guide that will take them through the whole journey.

These pre-writing activities are offered as an invitation, as a menu of possibilities you may choose from to help you find your way into writing. Follow your natural curiosity and interest in choosing the ways into your story. And if something not mentioned feels helpful, do that!

Take Note

One great place to begin is by taking some notes about your birth experience. If you are pregnant or have recently given birth, plan to jot down or otherwise record some key details of your birth as soon as possible after baby arrives. If it's been a while, but you are intending to write soon, start recording your thoughts about what to include as they come in.

These notes do not need to be in narrative form; they may be better as bulleted lists or phrases, whatever naturally arises. They can be written—in a notebook, scratch paper, sticky notes, a whiteboard, a napkin—or recorded in another way. Smartphones can be great allies in our early writing process. Our contributor Kelsey says, "I often have phrases or lines that pop into my head prior to finally sitting down to write it all out, and I try to jot those down so my mama-brain doesn't forget them. Siri [an iPhone voice recognition program] has recorded many a random thought of mine!"

While we women have impressive recall when it comes to our experiences of birth, we inevitably lose track of some of the details as they fade in time. Do your best to write down the more specific details of your experience that you wish to capture. See the box below for more ideas about what to take notes on in the early days (or as soon as you decide to write your story).

What to Jot Down After Birth

- Any contextual details you can recall:
  Day of the week, time of day
  Weather
  Sensory details (smells, sights, sounds, tastes, etc.)
  Names of birth support team
  Focal points

- Chronology—the facts and timing of your birth's unfolding (consider sketching a simple timeline)

- Thoughts and feelings—what were you thinking and feeling at various points in your birth experience?

- What was said—by you and others

Sensory Markers

The use of memory markers can be of great benefit as you sit down to write your story.

Activate your senses—your sight, hearing, smell, touch, and even taste—as relevant to assist you in recalling your story. Eat the same meal you enjoyed in early labor or just after birth. Smell the same lotion, essential oils, or other scents you remember from this time. Listen to (or sing!) the same music (if you had a birth playlist, play that). Look through pictures of your pregnancy, birth, and/or early postpartum experience, if available.

It can also be helpful to return to a place where some or all of your birth story unfolded. You may not be able to saunter into the labor and delivery ward at your leisure with computer in hand, but you could go for the same drive you took to the hospital, or the same walk around the neighborhood you took in early labor. Go into the room in your home or the place where you labored before going to your birthing place.

Like smells, sights, tastes, sounds, and textures, places hold strong memories for us, and this may be a great way to jumpstart your memory and get the creative writing juices flowing.

Key Words

As mentioned earlier, the story skin speaks in nouns and verbs— the facts and the external action of your story.

The deeper layers of muscle, connective tissue, and bones speak in adjectives—more nuanced, descriptive of, and connected to the inner landscape of our experience.

To begin to dig beneath the surface facts into the emotional terrain of our tale, complete this simple exercise.

JOURNAL ACTIVITY

If you could use only three words to describe your birth, which of the following three words you would use? (Feel free to use words not on this list.) Take it a step further by explaining why you chose each word.

Afraid	Healing	Scary
Awe-inspiring	Heart-Opening	Scattered
Challenging	Heart-wrenching	Shocking
Chaotic	Incredible	Slow
Coherent	Indescribable	Spiritual
Connected	Intense	Supported
Confused	Joyful	Terrifying
Determined	Life-altering	Traumatic
Difficult	Lonely	Trusting
Divine	Loud	Unbelievable
Ecstatic	Loving	Uncentered
Empowering	Overwhelming	Unforgettable
Fast	Painful	Vulnerable
Focused	Peaceful	Wonderful
Grateful	Quiet	
Hard	Respectful	

Key Questions

Sometimes it can help to begin fashioning our stories with a mind for what is most important about them. Seeing the forest for the trees, so to speak. Why are we writing our stories in the first place, and what is most important about our experience of giving birth?

To that end, the following questions can be used as short writing prompts to help you begin framing your story by what is most essential to you. Answer any or all of the following questions in a journal.

JOURNAL ACTIVITY

You may wish to meditate, dance, go for a walk, or any other activity to get the creative juices flowing prior to answering these key questions. Give yourself a time frame, maybe ten to twenty minutes, to complete each prompt. Your responses may or may not make it directly into your story, but they will certainly influence what you have to say and how you feel about it.

- What is your strongest memory from the birth experience?
- If you could change one thing about your birth experience, what would it be?
- What has changed in you as a result of this birth?
- If you could tell others one piece of wisdom you gained from your birth experience, what would it be?
- What did you receive in your birth experience that you might not have otherwise ever received?
- What of your old life died in the birth process?
- What is one thing you are afraid to say or write about your birth experience?
- What really matters about your birth?
- What does your birth experience have to do with the rest of your life?

Use the Guide

If you are enjoying using specific questions to call up the details of your birth experience, consider using the more detailed Birth Story Guide offered in Appendix C. These questions will take you from pre-conception to parenthood. It can be a great tool to journey through each part of your experience in a non-intimidating way and can be an excellent place to begin.

Create a Map

Another way into your birth story, especially if you are a more visual person, would be to create a map of your story (which could also be described as a timeline or scene sketch). This is a process of mapping out your story using the concepts from Chapter 9: Birth Story Narrative Arc and Chapter 10: The Birth Story Layers.

JOURNAL ACTIVITY

Take out a piece of paper—you could use regular-sized printer paper or go big and opt for a poster board (I prefer the latter). Orient the page to landscape, with the width greater than the length. From left to right on the top, in five columns, write the words: EXPOSITION, RISING ACTION, CLIMAX, FALLING ACTION, RESOLUTION. Under each, you may make notes about what each of these elements will contain for you. Then under that, make three rows, noting on the left: SKIN, MUSCLES, BONES and noting what each of these layers of the story includes (see example). Now that you've set up your map, fill it in as relevant to you. Use the table on the next page as an example to guide and inspire you.

LAYER	EXPOSITION Hook	RISING ACTION	CLIMAX	FALLING ACTION	RESOLUTION
	Backstory, frames, lenses, influences	Labor	Birth	After Birth	Integrate experience into life
SKIN scenes facts what when where	past due non-stress test & ultrasound deciding when/ how to intervene crying over lunch	birth center office visit watching movies with husband & pasta dinner active labor through the night vocalizing through each contraction drive to birth center	going to birth center getting into the tub meditation music surrouned by midwives & birth assistants cold sunny winter morning, a Wednesday	from tub to bed hemorrhage painful uterine pushing eating pizza learning how to nurse getting stitched up	early days back home
MUSCLES key thoughts & feelings relationships central characters major dialogue	READY impatient worried uncomfortable discouraged "why won't my body cooperate?" kindness of midwife	at peace with labor progression staying present for each contraction feeling connected to partner & doula	WOW! super intense feelings moving into the timeless reality of Labor Land not hearing anyone	exhaustion still deep in another dimension neutrality at the bleeding looking at daughter felt cozy and cared for	transformed to creature called Mother awe for the body interdependence between child and me looking at her for hours; it never gets old
BONES making meaning symbols	learning surrender & trust letting go of expectations & surrendering	total trust & presence oneness deep connection to father primal nature	creative divine feminine bringing me to spirit door to collect my daughter WOW	attention on my new role allowing myself to be supported the art of receiving faith & trust	heart-bursting mother love connection to instincts power of the feminine feeling unsure & unsteady

Now, this is a pretty linear map, like the clean grids of a city's streets. You may wish to create a less linear map of your experience, perhaps resembling more of a forest or rural place. Perhaps you scatter your key words on a large piece of paper and create clusters around each with facts, thoughts, feelings, and lessons/meanings for each. Maybe it's a Venn diagram, maybe it resembles a subway map, maybe a pirate's map to the ancient treasure, where X marks the spot. However you are called to do so, make this map your own. And then use it as a guide to create the narrative tale of your birth experience.

Meditation

Yet another way into your story is to meditate on your experience, visualizing the story before you sit to write it. I offer a meditation in Appendix D at the back of this book. There is some overlap between this meditation prompt and the guide; feel free to use either or both in support of your process.

Movement

As a Qoya, yoga, and movement teacher, I value the importance of moving the body as a way to influence the mind and to explore and express the truth of our experiences.

In this context, movement can be a great way into your story, to get the creative juices flowing and connect you to the energy and essence of your birth experience. After all, your birth story happened in your body. Why not connect with it intimately before calling on your mind to record its experiences?

This may be as simple as putting on your favorite song and dancing however it feels best for the next five minutes. It may be a simple sequence of your favorite yoga poses. Perhaps you hold a restorative pose for ten to twenty minutes in silence before you write. (Consider reclined supported butterfly pose, or *supta baddha konasana*.) You might also go for a walk or run (the latter not recommended in the early postpartum). Please see Appendix E for a Qoya-based movement ritual you may use prior to writing. It gives you a beautiful container in which to connect to the birth energy (through breathing and visualization), to shake out anything holding you back from writing your story, and to express the story of your birth through movement as a portal into the writing process.

Because, through movement,
we remember.

CHAPTER FOURTEEN

Removing Writing Blocks

The worst enemy to creativity is self-doubt.
SYLVIA PLATH

———————————

WHILE MANY OF THE EXERCISES ABOVE are intended to help you avoid the potential roadblocks along your writing path, you may still discover some stubborn stones along the way. Here are some of the most common writing blocks I've encountered in those I've coached through this process . . . and how to get through them.

"I don't have enough time."

There are a million things we could do besides writing our birth stories, which means we can easily muster a million excuses.

Mamas have a lot on their plates, always in our mothering days but especially postpartum. Early on, we are exhausted, adjusting to the wild world of Babyland, learning how to feed and cater to another being's every need, healing, and the list goes on. After many years, we still find our plates delectably full—with activities, balancing motherhood and womanhood, meeting many people's vying needs, and taking care of ourselves.

So yes, all of this is true. It can be helpful to write down (or speak into a voice-recording program) all the reasons you don't have time to write. Let that be true. And then really question it.

If you really want to write, is it possible to take ownership of your desire and give yourself permission to meet it? What activities in your life could you exchange for a small spurt of writing time?

Maybe it's the twenty-minute zone-out on Facebook each night. Maybe it's reducing an hour of TV time at night to thirty minutes of TV and thirty minutes of writing. Maybe you lock yourself in the bathroom for ten minutes a day.

Where can you reclaim some of your time so that you can use it as you truly desire?

"I'm not a good writer."

> *Notice your reluctance to writing and why that is—are you*
> *caught up in the pressure to make pretty words? Have you*
> *ever considered yourself a writer? Are you overwhelmed by*
> *the events and don't know how to make meaning of them?*
> *Do you not have a forum for writing? What is holding you*
> *back? Notice why you are hesitating, accept that hesitation,*
> *and allow yourself permission to do it anyway.*
>
> KELSEY STARRS

"I am not a writer." "I am not a good writer." "Whatever I write won't be good enough." "I don't know how to do this." [Fill in the blank with your own similar statements]

Ooh, the inner critic inside of each of us can be such a &@>?! Our inner critic is that voice in our heads that tells us negative things, places limitations on our perceived abilities, and often discourages us from taking risks.

This is often a voice we have internalized from our childhoods. While she can be a real beast, she serves a purpose—her job is to try to protect us from the hurt we risk in feeling vulnerable and stepping out of our comfort zones.

I personally dance with my inner critic all the time in my writing. She tells me that I am not a good enough writer, that I don't have the right things to say, that people won't like what I say, that I am not qualified enough, etc.

Sometimes, her voice wins. She discourages me from writing, and I find other ways to fill my time.

One day, feeling particularly sick of rejecting and devaluing the writer within, I tried something new. I turned around (mentally), and I faced her dead on. With compassion. It was as if I said to her:

"Okay, I am listening. I am here. Tell me everything."

And then I let her have a bloody field day, feeding me all the reasons why I shouldn't and couldn't possibly write. Ooh, she can be nasty! I took it all in, scrawling it down in red Sharpie on an Icelandic newspaper (what I had in that traveller's moment), breathed deep, and asked her tenderly:

"What are you protecting?"

A quiet voice rose up inside, one that lives in my core, and I realized this cranky critic was devoted to sheltering *her*, this vulnerable, tender, sensitive, golden part of me. She wants so completely to be loved, seen, and accepted.

While vulnerable and tender parts don't suddenly toughen up when witnessed (they aren't meant to—there is great power in this aspect of our nature), just allowing my critic to be heard softened her enough for me to get past the blocks and get on with the courageous telling of my tale.

JOURNAL ACTIVITY

I suggest you do the same. Flip to the next free page in your journal and write about all the reasons you cannot and should not write your story. Really let your inner critic have her say. What is she afraid of? What is she sure is true? Let her spill it all. And then breathe it in and ask the question, "Inner critic, what are you protecting?" And let it just be. Notice in the following moments and days how your relationship to her messages shifts. My great hope is that you too will find a softening. She may not disappear, but she may no longer be running the show. Your wise, confident, true voice can now emerge and take the reins. Return to this exercise anytime you feel blocked in your process (or your life!).

"I am afraid to admit the truth."

Sometimes we can be afraid to look at our more difficult or darker experiences. We may believe that keeping them in the cellars of our minds will keep us safe from them. They cannot hurt us or anyone else if they are locked away down there. We are afraid that if we let them into the light of day they will tear us apart. The great irony is that it's quite the opposite. When we relegate the truth of our experience to the dim dungeons of our consciousness, we leave them undigested, unprocessed, and frozen in time. They become lodged in the river of our psyches, preventing the free flow of our creative life force.

Believe it or not, you have survived living through your experience.

You have faced the monster and you are still alive. Admitting the truth of your experience allows you to free yourself from the shackles, to process and digest your experiences, to reclaim every corner of the castle that is your life. (See Chapter 5: Writing to Heal.)

If you are afraid to write your experience, honor that feeling. What you've experienced has left you hurt, tender, vulnerable. Take your storytelling slowly. Write on your own terms. Call in all the support you need. Write yourself free. It is possible.

"I am afraid of what others will think."

How many times have we directed the course of our lives based on this internal detractor? This internal limiting worry has silenced many important voices and killed their chance of living out in the world, where they can be of service to their owner and others. This is one of the key reasons I am a huge advocate of writing for yourself first—allowing your voice to come out unscripted and uncensored so that you can touch the truth without hesitation or limitation.

Sometimes we think our writing is only worth doing if it is to serve someone else. Maybe we want to write our stories for our children or for our community. Writing purely for ourselves can feel selfish or unworthy of our time.

So much of mothering asks us to consider others' needs when choosing how we conduct our lives. For many generations, the cultural creed for mothers has bordered on martyrdom. As humans, women, and especially mothers, we dance this two-step between our needs and the needs of others. In the case of writing your birth story, give yourself full permission to write first for yourself and only for yourself. This process is for you. Sure, it may eventually be for your partner or child, or perhaps your community and even the world—but first, let it be for you.

In the face of this fear, I invite you to sit in compassion with this internal voice. And then carry on with the writing of your story. Reach out for encouragement from the trusted kin around you; let them mirror for you the permission-granting you need, if necessary.

Write for yourself. Let that be enough.

If and when you choose to share, may you feel great courage and power in telling the truth of your experience, regardless of what anyone else thinks. Everyone else's opinions are their business. Your business, your duty, is to your own inner sense of the truth. Pledge allegiance to your soul voice—it's the only voice that really matters.

Let's get writing.

CHAPTER FIFTEEN

Writing the First Draft

Writing is physical and is affected by the equipment you
use. In typing, your fingers hit keys and the result is block,
black letters: a different aspect of you may come out. I have
found that when I am writing about something emotional,
I must write it the first time directly with hand on paper.
Handwriting is more connected to the movement of the heart.
Yet, when I tell stories, I go straight to the typewriter.

NATALIE GOLDBERG

AFTER YOU HAVE COMPLETED THE PRE-WRITING EXERCISES that inspire and support you best, with what tools will you choose to write your story?

Will you press the red record button on your iPhone as you tell your mirror, baby, or best friend the tale of your birth, then transcribe this story later? Will you grab your child's crayons and scribble away on a huge writing pad? Will you be scratching out a first draft on airplane napkins? (Hey, young babies often sleep on airplanes—just saying.) Will you write in a journal? Will you type on the computer? Your smartphone? My suggestion is to write with the tools that motivate you to tell your story.

Tools for the Job

If given the luxury of choice, consider writing some or all of your story by hand first. Consider at least making notes about the birth experience by hand as soon after the birth as possible. If you wish to type your story, as many do with good reason, print out your words so you can touch them, see them, and read them off screen and on paper.

Let your words take a physical form.

Junk Journal

When we set an intention to begin writing, we may be tempted to go out and buy a shiny new journal and fancy pen. But then it sits there, unopened and unapproachable. Why? Because this new "perfect" journal doesn't mirror the messy story, scribble of thoughts, and lived experience of our stories; it also doesn't give us permission to be "imperfect" in our storytelling.

Consider going to the dollar store or supermarket, or digging into an old stash of notebooks, and find a journal that has been well loved or is simply ordinary and unadorned. Beat it up a little. Then write.

Let It Flow

> *A story has no beginning or end: arbitrarily one*
> *chooses that moment of experience from which*
> *to look back or from which to look ahead.*
> GRAHAM GREENE

All first drafts are about getting thoughts on paper. When you first write, give yourself permission to just go with the narrative as it arises in your mind. Don't concern yourself with getting it "perfect"—

saying it in just the right way, using correct punctuation, or any of that. Kindly tape shut the mouth of your cranky inner critic. Dismiss the English teacher in your mind. The best way to start is to just begin at your beginning and write until the end without permitting any voice but your heart's narrator to speak.

That said, don't worry about writing in chronological order of how things happened if that's not working for you. Begin where you are compelled to begin. If that is when you first conceived, start there. If it's when the baby is crowning, or what happened yesterday, that is fine too! It's okay to miss some details or even whole "stages" of the story—you can go back and fill them in later. Whatever happens, don't let yourself get stuck somewhere. If you do encounter a roadblock, don't falter; just move around it and keep writing. Just write and keep writing until you are done.

Be Authentic

Let the real, true you speak through your birth story. Honor all of your story, not just the pretty parts. Give yourself permission to write about everything that happened (and maybe didn't happen) and how you felt about it all. If there are painful moments, write about them. Those moments of deep vulnerability are the richest elements of your story.

You may have other people's versions of the story in your head at this point. Maybe you know already how your partner felt when the baby crowned, or how your midwife described your active labor, or what your photographer thought was the most touching moment of your birth. Don't let those voices distract you or hinder you from expressing how you thought and felt throughout your journey. It requires great skill to listen for your instrument amid the symphony, but you must if you are to play well.

Don't feel like you have to sound a certain way. If you want to be funny, be funny. If you want to be serious, be serious. Want to be poetic? Let loose, Dickinson. If you are normally a straightforward person, tell your story matter-of-factly. If you cuss like a sailor, drop a few F-bombs in there. Let it be you, through and through. Don't feel like you have to conform to the genre. Be yourself and write it as it comes naturally. Give yourself permission to be funny, wacky, serious, whatever feels right to you.

Dustin's story below is such a shining example of how great a story can be when we let the full light of our personality shine through our writing.

DUSTIN'S STORY

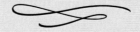

"Honey, can you *please* wake up and time my contractions?"

That's my wife. And the way she said the word *please* indicated to me that this wasn't the first time she'd asked. It also explained a very strange dream I was having in which a honey badger was asking me to wake up and time his contractions.

I reached for my phone and hit the shortcut I had created to go straight to the stopwatch feature, bypassing two extra buttons a woman married to a lesser husband might have to endure. I'd been ready for this moment my entire life. And by that, I mean I had sex once nine months ago.

I diligently timed my wife's contractions for the next few hours until my notes said it was time to get the turkey out of the oven. I called the doctor's office, followed the number tree to "If this is a labor emergency, press...", and left a message with the understanding that the on-call physician would call back within twenty minutes.

"Um, hi. My name is Dustin Fisher, wife of Jennifer Morrison. I mean, she's my wife. And she's been in labor for a couple hours, and the contractions are less than five minutes apart now. And, um, please call me back soon. Thanks. Oh. My number is 443-555-3077, or you could call my wife—*what's that, honey?*—okay, call me please. Thanks, and I look forward to talking to you soon."

Our doctor called back ten minutes later and told us to come into the hospital to labor there. My wife and her sister, who was visiting from Texas for just this reason, grabbed their go-bags and headed to the car while I packed mine. Something I'd meant to do weeks ago. The reasons I hadn't bothered to do this yet—a task that could possibly take as little as seven minutes—will be covered in future therapy sessions. I attempted to remember the list of things I made, most of them being props for photo ops to show the internet how cool a dad I was already. Cameras, socks, and mini-footballs were tossed haphazardly into a Giant grocery bag as I was being yelled at from downstairs to *just hurry the fuck up, you should have done this weeks ago!* I learned later that in my haste, I threw in a light bulb and my *Monk* bobblehead, both of which are surprisingly useless in childbirth.

It was 5:00 in the morning when we got going. I had printed out directions to Sibley Memorial Hospital from my work, from her work, from our old apartment, and from our new house, which we had moved into twelve days ago. This is my version of prepared. Mind you, I hadn't yet tested any of those routes—something I meant to do weeks ago.

I had assumed we would just take my Civic, but Jenn's sister had come in a minivan, and the both of them had just assumed we would take that. I was told in no uncertain terms to *just figure it out.* So I decided to drive a big van with a couple huge blind spots that I'd never driven before to a place I'd never been before for the most important commute of my life.

We got into the car, and Jenn's sister plugged in her GPS in a sisterly attempt to make things easier. The TomTom and the printed directions immediately started arguing with each other about whether to go through or around D.C. *Oh, come on! I do NOT have time for another argument right now!* I decided to venture into the city with the printed directions despite the very irritated British lady recalculating at every intersection.

About halfway there, I began to question the leadership of Google Maps and my ability to properly interpret the complex directions to get around the Convention Center. Washington, D.C. is laid out almost completely like graph paper, with perpendicular, intersecting roads pointed exactly due north, east, west, and south with some notable—and on this morning, unfortunate—exceptions. I was off the grid. So I turned TomTom back on and waited for her take on things to hopefully get me back on track. *Turn right*, she says. I'm not buying it. That's the wrong way. But I do it anyway. *Turn right again.* OK, TomTom! You picked a bad time to get all sensitive about our earlier disagreement. So I reached for a third opinion, my very detailed map of D.C. that I keep wedged between the seats of the car. Of the Civic. Back at the house. Now firmly butting up against pissed off, I shut TomTom back off, crumpled up my Google Map, and navigated my way through D.C. by memory/logic/blind luck.

While driving in crisscross patterns through the city, I started to question my preparedness for this moment. *Why hadn't I practiced this route yet? Why hadn't I packed my go-bag? Why haven't I read any of the eighty-seven books that were handed down to me about raising a child? Is this not what I want? Is there still more I feel like I need to do before I have a child? Am I too selfish to have a child?* Maybe I got myself caught up in expectations and I wasn't ready to be a parent after all.

We somehow got to Sibley Memorial Hospital around sunrise. At 6:15 a.m. Jenn and I were shown to a maternity room. The nurse checked Jenn's cervix. Not dilated. No epidural.

Our birthing plan originally had an *epidural-if-necessary-but-preferably-not* clause in it. After a ceremonial handing-down of baby gear at a dinner with some parent friends, the mother said that she was on the same plan. Once the pain pushed her passed the if-necessary part, she got an epidural. She agreed right there on the spot to have a second child before even birthing the first one. *Shit. I can do this.* That is the power of an epidural. And so our plan turned into *epidural-likely*.

The pain came from somewhere in the neighborhood of left field. 6:47 a.m. was the contraction I made note of, the Holy Shit moment of the labor. Her grip tightened, her face tightened, and her uterus tightened. It was time to implement the *epidural-likely*.

Still not dilated, still no epidural.

We decided to walk around the hospital to force the issue. Less than thirty seconds later, we were back in the room. I was told to rub Jenn's shoulders harder to distract her from the pain. I was then waved off and asked to get out of her way.

Jenn was desperate for some sort of pain management, and we hadn't gone to any Lamaze classes. All I knew about Lamaze was Bill Cosby's stand-up routine, and I had been told almost daily in the month leading up to this date that I wasn't allowed to be funny. She shushed me at one point after an attempt at lightening the mood with humor (the reason she married me). That *shhh* sound became her Lamaze. Every contraction was accompanied by several shushes repeated at different volumes, frequencies, and durations which indicated the amount of pain she was in. Like a cricket's chirps. The quicker, louder, and the more painful the contraction, the harder I would massage her.

The ones when the words *shit shit shit* would come out were the worst. We created a more effective language between us than when we speak to each other.

8:00 a.m. Shift change. The new nurse couldn't find the cervix opening either. She said it might be behind the baby, whatever the hell that meant. Sounds to me like the bowl being behind the soup. Also of note is that this lady, however honorable her intentions, had extremely long fingernails, which were aggravating an already extremely aggravated woman. There is probably no other profession where having short fingernails should be more of a requirement. Maybe a knuckleball pitcher. The presence of this nurse, however painful for my wife, thankfully alleviated my status as scapegoat for the time being.

The doctor came in around 8:30. The cervix was still closed. "You know what they say. A watched cervix never dilates." Sure, *she's* allowed to be funny. But this lady had her shit together. Apparently we were super effaced (my interpretation of what she said) and something about a station that sounded promising despite not being dilated. It was almost as if the cervix was sewn shut. "Mrs. Morrison, have you ever had a procedure done that might have scarred your cervix?"

Seriously!? How has no one even brought this up yet? Eight months of doctor's visits and four hours of painful contractions with the entire medical staff under the belief that this was the most complicated uterus they'd ever seen. And that's the answer? "Oh, well, that may be what's going on here. Let me see if I can get my finger—oh, yeah. There she goes. Wow. Up to three centimeters already. Oh, and I broke your water, but you probably figured that out already." Oh yes, I did. Hey, how about that epidural now, you idiots?

It was 12:15 p.m. We had been in the hospital for six hours now and were starting to see some progress for all our efforts. That sadly was about to stop. Jenn was comfortable and smiling for the first time since we got here—sitting back in her motorized chair, sipping a margarita, and humming "Cheeseburger in Paradise." After two hours, the nurse said we were fully dilated and had a +2 station [referring to the location of baby's head in mom's pelvis], and Jenn took some Maalox-type stuff for her stomach. We started to push on every contraction. The contractions at this point had to be pointed out to Jenn from a monitor, as she could no longer feel anything, including her left leg, which I was assigned to hold in the air this entire time. And so we tried. Very unsuccessfully. After half an hour of this, we decided to sit back and "labor down," which is doctor-speak for taking a break.

I started doing some research. Who would our daughter share her birthday with? What famous people were born on June 21st? It was a depressingly abysmal list. Juliette Lewis and Wade Phillips were among the most popular. And Meredith Baxter. Wait. Michael Gross, too? So both parents from *Family Ties* were born today? And they're both turning sixty-five? That's got to be a misprint.

At 3:35, the nurse came back in and suggested we start again. Jenn still couldn't feel anything. Considering what we had gone through at 8:00 a.m., that was a decent alternative, but now she was trying to push this thing she couldn't feel.

Like reaching through an empty window and blindly shoving air, and shoving it as hard as you can.

Toward the end, I saw a shift in Jenn's modesty. In the beginning, she had her sister hold a blanket up while the nurse was checking for dilation so that I couldn't see. Me. The guy that did this to her. When it was finally go-time after ten hours, she was waving in the catering staff.

What happened next is often referred to as a miracle. I don't know that I'd go that far. However, the fact that something that large and alive can come out of another human being is quite impressive. Nice job, Nature. But I'll reserve the term *miracle* for something that doesn't happen 490,000 times a day. Like Franco Harris catching a ball off a defender's helmet, for example.

Jenn was physically and emotionally spent, and I was thrown up on at one point, but at 4:28 p.m. on the summer solstice, Mabel Michelle Fisher was born, a healthy baby to two healthy parents, one of them crying slightly more than the other.

Offer Details and Engage the Senses

The best birth story-writing makes us feel like we are looking over the shoulder of the birthing woman as she bravely brings her baby into the world. To invoke this feeling, we need lots of details. When we write this way, our memory comes alive; the story we write is richer and more valuable to us with the passage of time and the inevitable fading of these details from our memory. It keeps our memories alive for us in a way that the brain simply cannot.

Writing with accurate and concrete detail is also one of the characteristics of a healing narrative. In fact, the more detail, the greater potential for healing. Do your best to include as many details as you can in your first draft, but don't get stuck on trying to include everything. You can always go back and add details later.

You may discover that certain parts of your story feel powerful to you, and you want to develop this scene as much as possible. I suggest slowing down that scene in your mind.

JOURNAL ACTIVITY

Write in your journal a short descriptor of the scene you want to amplify and then list the senses: SIGHT, SOUND, SMELL, TASTE, TOUCH.

Next, brainstorm what was coming through each sensory channel during your experience. Here is a partial example of what this journal activity could look like:

"When I first held my baby"

SIGHT:

• Her squishy wet face, red and crying
• Her tiny wrinkled shoestring-fry-thin fingers with their long fingernails
• Her soft, thin brown hair and the tiny little covering of brown lanugo around her face and down her back
• Her long eyelashes, like the legs of a "daddy longlegs" spider

SOUND:

• The calm, loving voice of her father cooing at her over my left shoulder
• The midwives, confidently assuring me this distressing cry is a sign of health
• The laughter of the doula and the photographer rejoicing at this new life
• The shrill cries of this new baby, strong-lunged and telling us all about it, like she would continue to do from this day on

TOUCH:

• Fresh, squishy skin covered in a clear fluid; the softest skin I've ever touched
• Warm bathwater holding me from the mid-torso down
• Comfortable air on my head, neck, shoulders, and chest
• The feel of the crisp woven receiving blanket wrapped around her, half dangling in the water

Don't Just Report; Reflect

We've talked a lot about this already, so I won't belabor the point. This is the idea that it is not enough just to stick to the facts of your story; you need to discover and disclose your inner landscape and the deeper meaning behind your experience. See Chapter 10 for more about the deeper, more reflective layers.

Put simply, when you write about something big in your story, take a moment to reflect on how you did or do think and feel about it. When you get toward the end of your story, you may want to reflect on the whole of your experience and what it means to you. Return to Hope's story on page 130 for a great example of how to weave reflection into your story.

Use Dialogue

It is not necessary to use dialogue, but it can be great to include, particularly when something someone said during your labor really stands out to you. It can also serve to develop the characters in your story, break up long stretches of narrative, add interest, convey tone and emotion, and contribute to the vividness of your tale.

Several story contributors in this book use dialogue to accomplish all these things and even reveal the deeper layers of their birth story. Consider Kelsey's use of dialogue in her story (on page 141):

> "What are you feeling?" she asked me.
> "I feel my babies. I feel my love for them, my overwhelming love for them. It's flooding every fiber of me and giving me courage and strength. I feel my love for Samuel. I feel my love for Geneva. And I feel my love for Miriam. They've come to me here, and I'm holding them. I want to hold them and cherish them and pour every ounce of myself out in love for them. It hurts so good."

She later admits she didn't actually say out loud any of the heart-stirring words she uses in quotes here, but she uses this device nonetheless as a way to get to the direct truth of what she was thinking and feeling in that moment. This dialogue gives us a glimpse into her inner landscape during this potent moment in her story.

Betsy, whose story appears on page 15, uses dialogue like a boss. Consider the effects of her opening alone:

> "The doctor said my water broke."
> The other end of the line was silent.

> *"Butch, you there?"*
> *"Yes." It was my husband's voice, but it was much quieter than I was used to.*
> *"Is he sure?" Butch asked, barely audible.*
> *"Of course, he's sure!" I said. "He said to call you and let you know they are admitting me to the birthing center. Do you remember where it is?"*
> *The other end of the line was quiet again.*
> *"I don't think I can drive," he said. "I think I'm going to be sick."*

Consider how much Betsy reveals to us about Butch and their dynamic in this brief dialogue and how this detailed account of their conversation brings you right into the story.

Several other contributors to this book also employ dialogue, which is worth exploring if you're curious about other ways it can be incorporated into your story. Nick, for example, uses dialogue in his story below to capture the more medicalized feel of the operating room.

NICK'S STORY

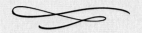

As my wife is wheeled away, I am left to pace.

And worry.

Everything will be okay. After all, I've been here before. Twice. But that knowledge still doesn't make it any easier.

This singular experience is the most nerve-racking one of my life. All the questions you never let yourself entertain. What if there are complications? Where would the kids go? How could I carry on?

The minutes drag on, feeling like hours as I wait for word that I can see her again. I don't want to miss this. I don't want there to be any trouble. I want to see my wife.

And my child.

Just when I'm ready to bust down the doors and demand they let me see her, make them prove to me that she is okay, there is a knock. A doctor in full surgical scrubs greets me with a smile. "We're ready for you, Dad," she says. "All the prep went fine, and your wife is waiting for you."

And with that, we take the long walk back to the operating room. I don my mask as the doors to a perfectly white room slide open, and I see her again. My heart jumps. She is laid on a table, a curtain clamped over her chest, cutting her in half. The stool waiting near her head is reserved for me, and as I take it, she smiles up at me.

I grab her hand and tell her she's doing great.

Now as the doctors set to work, monitors beeping, activity buzzing just out of sight, my stomach tightens again. I know this is it, the day we've been waiting for, the moment of truth.

And yet, for any worries I have, I'm not the one going under the knife. I'm not the one who has been doing all the work for this these last nine months.

She asks for something to calm her feeling of nausea, and I'm back to reality. I can see her lying there, arms spread, and I smile again and say how proud I am of her, tell her what a great job she's doing and how excited I am.

From behind the sheet, I catch snippets.

"Can I have a little suction here?"

"Clamp."

"Are you ready?"

"How does that look?"

Then my wife says it feels like there's a rock sitting on her sternum. Her anesthesiologist peeks over the curtain and smiles. "Sure thing, that rock's name is..." and I can see the nurse sitting on my wife's chest give him an ugly look. Shortly after, someone asks if we want to know what it is.

I look up to see a tiny baby boy in front of me.

"It's a boy!"

Kate is aware enough to smile up at me—we were both predicting a baby girl.

We talk for a minute, and then I can't take the wait any longer. "I'm going to go get a good look at him," I tell her. A squeeze of her hand and a kiss on her forehead, and soon I'm looking down at a different beautiful face, one I've been waiting to meet for nine months.

As the surgeons take care of my wife, the nurses around me give my new son a thorough once-over.

Weight.

Oxygen levels.

Heart rate.

Breathing.

Color.

Then, "Would you like to cut the cord?" And as I am handed the scissors, it sets in: I'm a dad again, and it's amazing.

Finally, baby and I make our way over to my wife, and he is placed on her chest.

Skin to skin.

This moment. *This* is what I've been waiting for.

CHAPTER SIXTEEN

Writing about Trauma

T HERE IS A PARTICULAR METHOD OF WRITING that researchers and writers have found to be most instrumental to healing trauma. Psychology professor and author James Pennebaker and his colleagues have conducted several studies over the past two decades about the healing power of writing.

In one of his studies, he and his colleagues split the study population into three groups. They all wrote about a traumatic experience, but the first wrote only about what happened, the second only vented about how they felt, and the third wrote about what happened and how they felt about it, then and now. This study showed a significant increase in physiological and psychological well-being only in the third group.

To use writing as an agent of healing, one needs to talk about what happened, how they felt about it at the time, and how they feel about it now.

It is this linking of events and feelings that provides therapeutic potential. This process supports integration of the emotional, linguistic, and logical aspects of our experience, activating both hemispheres of the brain for a more holistic processing of the event. Describing what happened, how we felt then, and how we feel now is a simple yet powerful healing technique. It allows us to track our inner world through time, and it charts our changing inner landscape.

Though I am unaware that Pennebaker makes this link, this method is the heart of Non-Violent Communication. NVC is an approach and philosophy that values recognizing and understanding our feelings and needs in order to increase deep, empathetic, conscious, and authentic connection with ourselves first, and then with others. Thus, in Appendix F, I offer a writing exercise that follows a process central to Non-Violent Communication, which is meant to help you digest some of the more challenging or charged aspects of your birth experience.

In addition to linking events and emotions through writing, Pennebaker also found that writing in short, definable time blocks over a series of sessions works best. More specifically, his work has found that writing about emotionally laden experiences for fifteen to twenty minutes daily for four days can provide many health benefits, including decreased anxiety and depression and a boost to our immunity.

Switch Hands

One practice that may help individuals process traumatic experiences through writing is using one's non-dominant hand to write their story (e.g. if you're right-handed, you'd use your left). This practice is thought to help one access their emotions in a different way than dominant-handed writing does.

You might experiment with using writing as a tool to process your experience over time. Often, for those of us with trauma, the one-and-done approach to writing is not as useful and therapeutic as using writing as a processing tool in conjunction with other sources of healing support.

Characteristics of Writing to Heal

• **Link events to feelings**
What happened? What did you feel at the time? Why? How do you
feel about it now? Why?

• **Find a balance between thinking and feeling**
Overly analytical and intellectual processing, and, conversely, purely
emotional venting about the negative aspects of an experience have
been found less effective than a more balanced approach to therapeutic writing. The key is integrating heart and mind wisdom and
enabling them to work as a team to serve you well.

• **Write in short successive sessions**
Writing in fifteen-to-twenty-minute increments over a period of four
or more successive days makes writing manageable and conducive to
positive outcomes.

• **Create order and organization**
The more accurate, concrete, and organized your writing (about
events, thoughts, and emotions), the greater the potential for healing.

• **Write in detail**
The more vivid, compelling, and specific the writing (as compared to
reflection that is vague or general), the greater the therapeutic potential.

• **Slow down**
Go slowly through the process of writing about charged or traumatic
events. Don't put any pressure on yourself to hurry; be patient with
yourself. When you get to a part of your story that holds pain or some
other charge, slow the telling down so that you can safely and fully
move through the process at a manageable pace. Know when to slow,
when to stop, and when to stay with your process. Use your feelings
as a trustworthy compass to guide you.

- **Invite in the Wise Witness**

Allow there to be a part of you that moves through this writing process as a witness. There can be that part that really feels and merges with all that comes up to the surface, but see if you can also connect to a part of yourself that can simply witness what is arising rather than getting caught up in it. Allow this wise witness to be a compassionate observer and companion as you wrestle with the truth.

- **Write a balanced emotional narrative**

The most healing narratives are those that not only explore the pain and challenges but also acknowledge the joys and pleasures present in the experience. Including the positive doesn't negate the trauma, but it does bring balance and a more complete representation of the experience. If you can't bring yourself fully into the "joys" of the experience, you may be able to express what sustained you during this time or what has sustained you since the event.

- **Stay open**

The most healing comes in writing when we are willing to hold our stories with an open hand: we aren't clenching so tightly that no light can get in, but rather we are willing to approach our storytelling with curiosity. We are willing to explore multiple angles or perspectives, open to new discoveries, and to look for the meanings in our tales (see the caveats of meaning-making on page 140).

- **Stay compassionate and kind**

As best you can, allow this process to be nurturing. Give yourself the compassion and kindness you would give a friend bravely going through this process of exploring trauma. As best you can, withhold self-criticism and judgment—about yourself, your experience, and your writing.

- **Don't force the process**

Always monitor yourself as you tread into the waters of trauma. The most important element of this process is to ensure your own safety and wellbeing. Carefully monitor the effects of your creative process on your wellbeing, and get help if/when you feel out of that safe zone.

• **Seek support**
When processing trauma through writing, I highly recommend working concurrently with a trained supportive therapist or other healing professional.

In Appendix G, I offer a number of shorter writing prompts that you may explore as you work through your story. You may find that they open up different understandings and explorations than what your mind has been running as its primary narrative. You may also re-visit Katie's series of writings on page 37, which are a great example of someone using short writing periods to process elements of her experience.

CHAPTER SEVENTEEN

After your First Draft

ALL SAID REGARDING THE VALUE OF WRITING AS A PROCESS, I'd say the majority of writers, of birth stories or otherwise, would prefer to consider their work complete after the first draft. It may be tempting to consider your story done after you type the last word, but some of the richest elements of story come in subsequent drafts, where we gain an even deeper understanding of what our experience is all about. They don't have to be major shifts; you may revise a sentence or two, clarify something, add more detail, take out something that doesn't ring true for you, or add some glimpses of your internal landscape at different points in your birthing journey.

Below is my invitation for how this process can look. As always, take what works and leave what doesn't. If something feels a bit uncomfortable, ask yourself, *is it pushing a healthy edge worth exploring, or does it really not work for me?*

Let It Sit and Breathe

When you are done with your first draft, Elsa that thing and *let it go* (you parents of a certain generation get the reference). Close the journal or the MacBook and let your story be, without looking at it for a couple days, a week, or longer before you return to it for editing.

Taking a break from your narrative will give you a fresh perspective when you return and enough space to see how you'd like to change it, if at all.

It's like making wine. All this love, care, and time are poured into the creation of this delectable nectar—the grapes are carefully picked, fermented, strained, aged in oak barrels in a cool basement, carefully crafted, and bottled. All this great work has unfolded to produce a masterpiece. And then the bottle is ready. But when it's time to open the bottle, you have to let the wine breathe before it will offer up its best flavors. The creation of your story is the wine-making. Letting it breathe once it's made—letting your story sit for a bit—is the way we can enjoy its flavors best.

Personally, whenever I write something, I am so close to it that I cannot really see it objectively. When I put it down, I create some space between us. When I return, I gain greater objectivity and can witness it in a way I could not before. I can see what works, what doesn't, what moves me, what doesn't, and sometimes I even discover something about myself by reading what I have written.

I sit with it for a few days to see what words, phrasing,
or composition come to me that I like better than
what I originally wrote. I know it's done when it feels
done—it's not science for me, it's an art informed by
intuition. I'm done when I feel the catharsis.
KELSEY STARRS

Reflect and Deepen

When you do come back to your draft, the first thing to do before changing a thing is to read it all the way through and reflect on the gestalt of it all. How do you feel about your story overall? Focus first on the content—what you have written. Anytime I read something I have written, I first read through it all once, resisting the urge to make any notations or focus on any specifics. I want to first feel my way back into the heartbeat of my story.

After you reacquaint yourself with your writing in this way, you can go back in and decide how to deepen your work. But first, before you figure out what you may wish to alter, appreciate what you love about what you wrote. What elements are strong? What words, phrases, sentences, sections move you? What feels inspiring? What feels really true?

From this place of honoring the work you've done so far, decide how you'd like to enrich your story. You might find that you desire to make one or more of these changes:

- **Revise:** Changing what is already there; this may be the way you say something, a word you use, a way you describe something, the emphasis on a piece of the story.

- **Reorder:** You may decide that you want to change the sequence of events or the descriptions or narrative about your experiences. Do you need to reorganize your storyline to strengthen what you've written?

- **Eliminate:** You may wish to cut what feels extraneous or what doesn't serve the whole of your work.

- **Add:** This is a great time to add details, fill in gaps, and add whatever feels like it is missing from your story. You may ask yourself: *What more can I say about this?*

- **Clarify:** Is there any way you can make what you have said any clearer? Are there parts that may be confusing?

- **Seek balance:** Look at how you have used positive and negative words to describe your experience. Anytime we use only the positive or only the negative to account for our experience, a red flag should go up because we are masking its complexity. A healing narrative offers both the positive and the negative. (I am thinking of an exercise I did on a writing retreat called "Yay. Boo." in which you write a story alternating between a "good" thing that happened and a "bad" thing that happened, revealing that interplay between positive and negative.)

- **Make connections:** Are there any places in your writing where you wish to link an event to your feelings about the event? Are there any connections to make between what you reveal in your story and other experiences you have had? Or to a common human experience?

During this phase of your creative process, focus less on the nitty-gritty, sentence-level issues of grammar, spelling, and punctuation, and more on the content and structure of your work.

Connect with Your Birth Support

You may choose to share your story or connect with others present at your birth as part of your drafting process. I recommend doing so *after* the first draft. If you start getting other people's voices and versions in your mind before writing, you may come out with a story that is made partly from your memory and partly from someone else's. (This is inevitable to some extent, of course, because we've often talked about our births or heard versions of them from others before we write.)

Dialoguing with a trusted support person can help you fill in possible gaps in your memory. Birthing women often enter the Labor

Zone, which is a universe existing one plane above and beyond the regular world—it is divine feminine territory. It can be hard after we leave this zone to reconnect with some of the things that happened while we were in it.

For example, I can't tell you what was said and hardly anything that was done around me after transition. I still ask my husband questions about this time: *Was I talking? Vocalizing? Quiet? What were the midwives saying to me while I pushed? What was our doula doing during this part? Where were you when this happened? Did they suction her when she came out? Did you get to catch her?* These are things I simply can't recall. I was in such a deep place in my labor, my body so exhausted that my mind simply didn't find it important to take in any of those details, yet I wanted to know them, and I wished to include them as part of my story.

Talking to someone who was part of your birth can help to fill in missing elements or add richness and detail to your story. But remember that you get to choose whether to add someone else's memories to your story. If it feels weird to add something that you don't remember or that doesn't feel part of your version of the story, leave it out. If you enjoy the details added by others and want to incorporate them, this is a great time to do so.

Consider Audience

Up until this point, I have urged you to write only for yourself and to pay no mind to concerns about who might read it and how you ought to write with them in mind. I stand by this through and through. However, many people will want to share their stories, and so here is the time we can consider audience in our writing.

The urge to censor seems only natural when we start to think about sharing because it's vulnerable to share our intimate truths, yet I urge you to be brave and authentic no matter your audience. If your mother-in-law reads things about your yoni that you'd never mention in the course of a dinner conversation, so be it. If your partner may feel sensitive in light of the way you characterized your early labor while he was away on business, but it feels true and important to your story, let your truth be known.

This encouragement aside, this is your story, and you are 100 percent in charge of the telling and the sharing of it. Maybe you are happy with this first draft version of your story in all its juicy truths. And perhaps you want to adapt this version slightly to share it with a broader audience. Having more than one version of your story is totally an option. (After all, many versions of our stories live in our hearts, why not the world?) Yet, I still encourage you to stand with the truth of your story in all its complexity and vulnerability.

Proofread

After you have reflected on your draft, made bigger changes in structure, clarity, or level of detail, and read with an eye for audience, this is the time when your inner English teacher gets to smooth out those grammar errors and misspellings should she so desire. Sometimes sentence-level issues can be hard to detect in our own writing. We have read them so many times that we tend to read them in our minds as we *intended* to write them, rather than how they actually appear on the page.

A few ways to illuminate these errors are the following. You can read your story aloud, to yourself, your little babe, the cat, another adult. Reading aloud can help you catch errors, run-on sentences, things that don't make sense, wordiness, and the like. If you really want to look at your story at the sentence level, you can read your story backward, one sentence at a time. Doing this sounds strange, but it removes the content from your consciousness so you can focus on the structure of your sentences. You may also choose to have someone else read your story and clean up your sentence-level issues.

All of this, of course, is optional. The grammar police will never come after you for errors in your birth story—this isn't a school essay and, really, grammar is not as important as content. But many of us are bothered by such errors and feel better when they are corrected, and for these folks, this is the place to clean it up!

Save It

This may seem obvious, but once you are done with your story, make sure to save it in a meaningful way. If you have typed your story, as many of us do, don't let it just sit on your computer. Print out copies. See your written words in tangible form. Read them on actual paper. Save a copy in your nightstand, in baby's book, somewhere special to you. If you want to go for the full gusto, make a cover for it (a great project for you crafty folk) and make it beautiful!

For some of us with harder stories to tell, it can also be really liberating to not save it. Rather, burning our story with an intention to release past hurts and move forward can be a powerful ritual. Do what feels right to you.

Write It Again

Remember that even if something is written, it is not written in stone. (That would be a lot of bother, anyhow.) You are free to change your story, how you feel about an aspect of your story, and what you think about your birth at any time. Your written account is a snapshot in time; it reveals something perfect and true at that moment—and it can be honored as such. Your story can always be revisited in your thoughts, in your words, in your writing, and in your heart.

As I mentioned above, I believe writing as a process is valuable, and many of us will benefit from writing our stories more than once as a way to explore and process our experiences further. For those who are open to using writing as an exploratory process for continuing to unearth the rare jewels from your experience, I include many additional writing exercises in Appendix G, including letter-writing, poetry, and more. These are fun and illuminating.

CHAPTER EIGHTEEN

Sharing Your Story

⎯⎯⎯⎯⎯⎯⎯⎯

ONCE YOU ARE DONE WITH YOUR STORY, share it if that feels right to you. Share it with your partner. Family and friends. Your birth team. Your child. Your mothers' circle. Share it on your own blog or contribute it to another person or organization's blog if you want to share your story with a wider audience. If you'd like to share your story with readers of this book and our online community, feel free to submit your story to us at JaimeFleres.com.

Though you never need to share your writing with anyone, sharing your birth story can be a powerful experience: it can facilitate connection with others, help other women and birthing families, aid your healing, and even influence the culture of birth.

Sharing to Connect

You may tell a tale that takes up residence in someone's soul,
becomes their blood and self and purpose. That tale will move
them and drive them, and who knows that they might do because
of it, because of your words. That is your role, your gift.
ERIN MORGENSTERN

Stories help us connect with other people. In our cantankerous culture where divisions between people—particularly women and especially mothers—are exaggerated, it's so refreshing and rewarding to read someone's birth story and see ourselves reflected in it. And we don't need to be women or mothers to connect with the birthing women in these stories. Birth stories are a brilliant metaphor for life at its truest. When we move beyond the "facts" of our birth and into the "truths" of our births, universal and timeless themes arise that all people everywhere can connect to in one way or another.

Sharing our birth stories with our partners and other support people can help them gain insight into our perceptions of the birth, which can increase empathy and understanding and invite dialogue about aspects of the shared experience. We sometimes assume that because a person was present they understand how it was for *us*, when really, they only know how it was for *them*. Sharing our stories with one another can help to illuminate how the experience was felt differently; we learn what moments were emphasized, which forgotten. A written birth story can be a vital tool for communication and understanding.

Sharing our story can also connect us with people who have shared similar experiences, and in this way, we may discover a support system beyond our family and friends. Sharing can have an unknown or unanticipated ripple effect. You never know how your story will help someone else.

Only experienced mothers and fathers can share certain truths about birth. While most women and men will underestimate or devalue their personal experience and wisdom about birth, they hold great keys to supporting other women and men through their experiences.

Dare to tell your story in a way that celebrates and values your experience and wisdom.

We can learn so much from each other, and our children will learn from us when we take the time to talk about our birth experiences.

Here, Vanessa writes about her birth with an intention and desire to share her experience and wisdom with other mothers.

VANESSA'S STORY

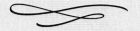

My labor began on Saturday afternoon, and my husband Jess and I went to the Durham community pool so I could float and relax. It was so peaceful and relaxing, having a weightlessness to soothe my tightening body. The contractions got a little stronger and stronger as the day went on. I called my midwife and my sister Jessica (who is also a midwife) so that they had a heads-up before bed. I drank a healthy glass of wine that evening to help calm my mind, and then I tried to sleep. I was so excited for the pending birth of our son and was hoping that these contractions were the "real thing," and I would have a baby in my arms soon.

I probably got about two hours of sleep that night when I woke up at 11:30 p.m. with a big ol' contraction. I then spent the next couple of hours pacing up and down the hallway with Jess near me. I felt like movement was my friend and helped me cope. Jessica (who made the three-hour drive from Grass Valley to Chico a couple hours before) woke up and spent the following next few hours with me as my labor intensified, and Jess got some sleep. I walked around the kitchen and family room, got on my hands and knees, waving my butt in the air, sat on a yoga ball, and moved into every position imaginable. Noise was one of my main coping mechanisms . . . I made a lot of "ohhhhhhhhhhh's" and "awwwwwwwww's".

I remember feeling so safe knowing my sister was there by my side. I didn't really need anything in particular from her; just to know that she was there calmed me.

Later that morning my midwife Dena and her assistant Amber arrived, and by that point I was at least five centimeters dilated, if not more. At that time I was in the water tub, really in active labor. I noticed in the tub my contractions became spaced farther apart, so I used it for a little weightless pain management and then tried my best to pull myself from it. I wanted my contractions to be effective and thought the tub was holding them back. I also felt I had too much time to think about the pending contractions to come, instead of just being in the moment. It was definitely an internal conflict to remove myself from the soothing tub, but I managed to do so and trust my instincts.

I then labored in the bedroom on the ground on hands and knees, standing and holding onto Jess, squatting, on the toilet, etc. I was *all over the place!* Finally around 8:00 a.m. I felt urges to push. This was interesting to me because I couldn't feel the baby's head yet and thought that I would only feel the urge to push when he was ready to be born, but apparently you have to push the baby down the canal, and then you push the baby out—I must have missed that part of the birth ed class!

I "loved" pushing. It felt more like pain with a purpose. I pushed the baby down pretty quickly but then had a hard time pushing the baby out. Apparently, my midwives informed me later, they had never seen such a strong perineum before! It would not stretch and it would not tear. They called it the *perineum of steel.* This is *so* ironic because Jess was obsessed with making perineum jokes at birth ed class. Turns out he really didn't perform his duty of perineal massage as he should have.

So after crowning for over an hour and pushing for over two hours, Dena asked me if she could give me an episiotomy. By that point I was all for it! I knew I just couldn't push him out, and it wasn't because I was afraid; I just couldn't get him past this one point. I was one of the few episiotomies given in the home. My sister, who is a home-birth midwife, had never seen one done in the home. After the episiotomy, I pushed him out without a problem, and Jackson Austin Pitney was born at 10:46 on Sunday the 19th of August. I got to hold him immediately, cone-head and all! He was so wet and sweet, and I was in love instantly. The placenta was born shortly after with ease, and then Dena sutured my perineum.

My overall labor and delivery were better than I could have imagined. I'm not going to deny it: it was the hardest thing I have ever done in my entire life! But with that said, I have never felt so proud and empowered and in love before, either. I don't think I could have done it without the help of such a wonderful support team. They fed me sips of Recharge after every contraction and bites of yogurt periodically. They told me I was doing great, encouraged me, calmed me, and helped me to feel safe.

To all the pregnant mamas out there, I highly recommend that when you feel labor coming on, EAT AND SLEEP! It is the most physically demanding job you can imagine, and you need the nourishment and energy stores to rock it.

Also, don't hold anything back. Let go of it all, whatever "it all" may be. For me, it was expressing that I was feeling unsure if I could do it or not and asking for support. It was asking if I was safe and getting the reassurance that I needed. It was also asking if I could push, because I wasn't thinking it was a good time to push yet, but in fact it was an excellent time to push.

After the birth, baby Jackson, Jess, and I got to rest in bed for an hour. His breathing sounded a little too labored, and my midwives decided we should get him checked out, so we went to Enloe Medical Center. I am not going to pretend that this was an easy transition, because it wasn't. We knew we wanted to be safe and not sorry, so we weren't hesitating to transfer, but it was really hard to pack up and leave our home at that point. I was still covered in all the birth fluids and had just been sutured from the episiotomy. I was in an extremely sensitive emotional state and was holding my baby with oxygen on his face. We got to Enloe, and it turned out he had fluid in his lungs. They decided he needed CPAP [continuous positive airway pressure] to help him reabsorb the fluid.

We stayed for two nights in the NICU, then in the nursery. Since I didn't deliver there, we weren't given a room, and I literally slept on a reclining chair for those days. That was rough! But the good news was that he improved so much that we were able to go home that Wednesday afternoon.

Because of the breathing problems and his struggles to latch well with a nasal cannula, however, nursing got delayed a full day, if not longer, and he didn't get the nourishment he needed. He was also expending more energy to breathe than most newborns, all of which contributed to dehydration, and eventually he ended up getting jaundice.

We went home for a night to recoup and then were back at Enloe for two more nights to put our baby under the bili lights, a standard treatment for jaundice. Again, this was very difficult but had to be done because his bilirubin levels got dangerously high. We were finally discharged on Friday afternoon and had our first full day at home, and he began doing so much better! I began pumping around the clock (after every feeding) and supplementing at the breast with a little tubing set (Lact-Aid) with moms' milk that was donated to me from moms in my community.

This was a lot of work, but *so* worth it! Little did I know, there were many challenges to come with nursing that involved my milk supply, a tongue tie, an uncoordinated tongue movement, and poor latch. We ended up working through them all, and at six months, after the initiation of solids, we were able to establish a healthy, calm nursing relationship and have been nursing ever since.

To all the mamas-to-be, each of you will have your own amazing birth story to tell that will transform you in remarkable ways. Just remember to trust in this process and communicate your needs throughout. You *will* get through it, and just when you might think you can't go on any longer, the most incredible part is just around the corner. Take good care of yourselves and accept all the help you can get. Make sure you allow for help and don't hesitate to ask for it if it is needed. Your job is to be with your baby, and that is it!

Sharing to Heal

The act of writing itself can produce a profound shift, but taking it a step further can help us heal. Sharing our writing with someone else offers them the gift of witnessing our raw truth and our incredible humanity. It can be a powerfully cleansing and vulnerable step to simply admit our truth to a trusted someone else. It can also open up dialogue about our story.

Sharing our story with others cracks open the tightly bound scar tissue surrounding our trauma and allows the light to seep through. This light has the power to break up our story and dissolve the hurt inside. We can begin to see what is true for us, or what we *think* is true for us, and we gain the power to decide whether or not there is room for revision. We can be witnessed and then, in that space of being seen exactly as we are, we can then choose to rewrite or reimagine our stories if we wish. And it may not be our story that changes at all, but our relationship to it—and that is akin to mountain-moving.

Sharing with Our Children

My daughter *loves* to hear the story of her birth. At the age of three, Maia connects most with the version of my story that revolves around what we ate during her labor, what kinds of sounds Mama was making during labor and as she crowned, how she pooped on Daddy's T-shirt within fifteen minutes of her birth, and how she loved to nurse right away. But this story will evolve over time, and I look forward to the day that she can read what I have written about my experience birthing her.

Writing your story can benefit your babe in a few ways. For one, a mama's psyche deeply affects her child's in nuanced and sometimes unseen ways. A healthy mama who has processed her story may be more available to her child than a mama with unresolved issues she carries in an invisible suitcase through her daily life. No one sees them, but they weigh her down.

222 BIRTH YOUR STORY

Your written story can also benefit your child by being a keep-sake they can return to throughout their lives. They see that you cared enough about your own experience and their birth to write about it. Knowing about our births is part of knowing ourselves. Just as every society has felt a deep impulse, a deep longing, to know its origins, so too do we long to know how it was that we came to be—however we perceive it along the spectrum between perfect and imperfect.

You can also support your child's perception and beliefs about birth—what it is and what is possible. Your written story may also be a tool that helps them prepare for birth someday themselves.

This all said, I will offer you a small caveat and minor exemption to my "write uncensored" recommendations throughout this book. If you intend to share your story with your child as they grow up, might I suggest reading your story through the lens of a child and feeling it out? Children may hear stories about their birth and create from them deeply held beliefs about themselves and the world. (Of course, they do this in all kinds of ways through life and, for better or worse, we are bound to contribute deeply to their beliefs about themselves and the world no matter what we do—it's in our parental job description). But there is a distinction between how we need to process the tougher parts of our stories and the words we choose to share with our child about their birth experience.

As I detail in my story on page 149, my daughter entered the world hours before the close of my forty-second week of pregnancy. Waiting for what seemed like F O R E V E R for her birth was hard on me. And I have written about that. I also choose to take responsibility for my own experience of this perceived lateness and have used words carefully so not to convey any fault on her part or any anger towards her. I don't necessarily edit myself in any great way, but I am a bit more conscious about language use and how it will affect her as a listener. If you plan to share with your child, maybe you read through with them in mind and decide how you'd like to share your story with them as they grow.

JOURNAL ACTIVITY

Consider for a moment what you know about how you were born. Do you know the details? How were they shared with you as you grew up? Did your mother document the story in any way? Do you wish she had? What do you wish you knew more about your birth?

Sharing to Shape Culture

Women will starve in silence until new stories are created
which confer on them the power of naming themselves.
SARAH GILBERT AND SUSAN GUBAR

Stories have the power to shape beliefs, choices, lives, and whole cultures.

By stepping into our power, speaking our
truth, and having the courage to share
our lives with others, we heal and liberate
ourselves and invite others to do the same.

We also have the power to change the master narrative of birth in our culture, which in turn can shape how birthing families experience birth moving forward.

Writing and sharing your birth story can be a political act. It can be a way of saying, "Birth is important. The *women* who birth are important. *My* birth is important." Regardless of how you feel about your birth, putting words to your experience is a powerful way to show that your experience matters. Because it does.

When Not to Share

*Our stories are not meant for everyone. Hearing them is
a privilege, and we should always ask ourselves this before
we share: "Who has earned the right to hear my story?"*
BRENÉ BROWN

For all these great reasons to share, there is an equal number of reasons not to share, or to at least think through your motives and the consequences of sharing your story. Our birth stories are deeply personal accounts; they don't need to be shared in order to hold value. In our social-media-dominated culture, it can feel almost necessary or validating to share in a public sphere, yet this may or may not offer you the support and connection you seek. Here are a few caution signs that you may want to consider more closely before sharing your story with a wider circle (social media or otherwise):

• **The search for approval:** if your motive for sharing is simply for approval of your writing or your experience (you know, to get a bunch of likes, or have it published in a certain space)

• **To evangelize:** to preach to others that your way is the best way, and convince them to agree with your own personal perception of birth

• **You are still tender and vulnerable about your story:** We will always be vulnerable about our birth stories, to some degree, because our births are deeply personal. And yet we may open ourselves to additional wounding if our stories are not thoughtfully shared with regard for our audience and how they may respond.

- **Using birth story as a weapon:** This may sound weird and is certainly not applicable to all, but if you share your story with a particular person with the intention of harming them with your account, you may want to reconsider how, when, and why you are sharing. We can and should tell the truth about our experiences as a way to heal, discover, and mend ourselves *and* be compassionate and considerate of others we share with. This isn't to say that we shouldn't speak our truths even if some may not like it; this is all to say that some additional consideration may be warranted.

Writing your birth story is not about outcomes, how pretty the words are, who reads them, how many likes you get on Facebook, whether it's accepted by this blog or that anthology. It's about doing what will hold meaning for you and constructing this experience of birth into one that will change you for good and for the better.
KELSEY STARRS

Celebrate and Return

Regardless of what you do with your story after writing, or how you feel about your story and/or your writing, I invite you to take a moment to honor your achievements. You conquered all the roadblocks to writing.

You dared to write as a way to remember, process, claim, heal, and honor your valuable story of birth.

It's time to celebrate your efforts.

During this celebration, however private or shared, make it a point to set an intention to return to your story in the future. Perhaps you decide to return to it every year on your child's birthday. Maybe you read it to yourself when they are babies, read it to them when they are small, and read it together as they get older. You may also choose to read it before or during a subsequent pregnancy. You might read it after long, hard days of parenting, to remember how it all began, the power in your meeting, and that sweet little babe who is growing into their own. Holidays (Christmas, for example, is a great cultural ritual that celebrates the birth story) and other special family occasions might also be good opportunities to read and reflect on this important chapter in your personal and familial history. Birth is the beginning of everything, and it's important to celebrate and remember our creation stories.

I deeply honor your journey through this book and through the process of writing your birth story. Thank you for being here and for doing the incredible work of birthing and parenting. May you continue to parent and write with tremendous compassion, tenderness, patience, and love for yourself. May you always know how important you are, how much your stories matter, and how much we need your voice in the world.

Keep writing about what matters.

ACKNOWLEDGEMENTS

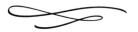

First and foremost, I'd like to acknowledge, honor, and thank my mother Christine for giving birth to me and for raising me—for all those precious little moments a child forgets or can't consciously access but will *feel* forever. Thank you, Mama, for your inextinguishable energy, love, and care.

To Billy, thank you for your love, support and encouragement. Just as you held my hand through our daughter's birth, so have you held my hand through every moment of life since the day I met you. Thank you for believing in me, for always encouraging me (especially when I'm in doubt), for supporting my dreams and passion for adventure, for listening to me talk about and read this book to you in various iterations 10,000 times, and for loving me through all that life has brought to us in the last decade. I am so grateful to have you in my life and by my side. Thank you for all that you are. I love you.

Thank you to each of this book's story contributors. Some of you I know intimately and some not well at all. Each of your stories lives in my heart. Thank you so much for sharing your stories. You are what makes this book brilliant. Thank you Alexandra Crosta, Nick Downey, Dustin Fisher, Jason Lew, Hope Lien, Katie Murphy-Olsen, Billy Mizejewski, Vanessa Pitney, Lauren Robbins, Lance Somerfeld, Kelsey Kreider Starrs, Aubrey Essex Wicks, Brandon York, Lindsay McKinnon, and Betsy Blankenbaker.

Thank you, Kate Hopper, you were the perfect editor for this project, and I am deeply grateful for you and our work together. Thanks for believing in this book and guiding its creation so wisely.

Thank you, Betsy Blankenbaker, for believing in me and my stories, for really seeing me when I needed it in Costa Rica, and for inviting me to France to finally honor the writer within. Thank you for your support and for your contributions to this book.

Thank you, Kelsey Starrs. Kelsey, this book would not be nearly what it is today without your brilliance, your love, your wisdom, your words, and your support. I am deeply grateful that I know you and for every moment I have spent with you. You are truly a soul sister and a vital part of this creation. If this book were a baby, you would totally be its fairy godmother.

Thank you to my dear friends Angela Vincent and Jessica Mairs for being some of the most amazing women I know and for supporting me through the drafting process with your expert birth professional and mothering eyes.

Thank you to Max Strom, who supported me through the early phases of this book; to Susan Shehata and Deb Rich for offering their expertise; to Lauren Lang for your editing support; to Amanda Coffin, my proofreader, for being an absolute joy to work with; to Emily Bohannon for your interior design work, to Ana Grigoriu for your exceptional cover design skills, to Gemini Adams for offering me your wisdom about publishing, to Danica Donnelly for lending your incredible photo and video gifts to this project, to Ali Rogers of PranaLens for your fantastic video artistry, and to all those who helped on the Kickstarter video project: Billy, Angela, Amy, Sophie, Kelsey, Alisa, Sarah, and Danica.

Thank you to everyone who supported the crowd-funding efforts on Kickstarter needed to make this book a reality.

Christine Maia-Fleres	Carrie Davies
Billy Mizejewski	Steve Dockendorf
LiYana Silver	Ryan Wheeler
Virginia Rosenberg	Alison Gray Gregory
Kelsey Starrs	Sarah Gottfried and Kaylynn Brown
Lindsay McKinnon	Tisha Reed
Betsy Blankenbaker	Janice Constable
Ryan and Kim Crawford	Fabiola Bergi
Tony Fleres	Tina Doellgast
Connie Fleres	Jessica Atkins
Lynda Woodman	Vanessa Pitney
Jim Dockendorf	Jeanette Beger

Cheri Schieck
Andrea Atherton
Steve Freeman
Joanie Lamb
Joyce Sellman
Suchi Sairam
Sue Kersten
Rebecca Wood
Katelyn Davis
Rosemarie Santoro
Jennifer Merritt
Jessica Mairs
Renee Delaney
Dana Whiddon
Carly Miyamoto
Claire Kohout
Erin Bergevin
Megan Brannan
Julie Sims
Samar Ciprian
Nadine Albuera
Marissa Bulris
Lyndsey Azlynne
Holly Palkowitsch
Amy Colwell Bluhm
Sarah Bach-Bergs
Rochelle Matos
Lance Somerfeld
Jamie Brazell
Ali Haeffner
Claire Garin
Amanda Coffin
Caylan Climpson

Kelly and Greg Carlson
Angela and Ben Vincent
Emily Berman
Ashley Brown
Micki Dirtzu Charley
Jackie Baker
Becky Bormann
Shannon Ledford
Rachel Mujerita MacDonald
Sara Ballard
Jen Quade
Danielle Coggins
Brook Holmberg
Cheryl Heitkamp/Willow Midwifery
Jeremy Korpi
Angie and Mike Sonrode
Katelyn Davis
Nicki Cullinan
Deb Dimino Kehoe
Kaci Florez
Jill Marie
Danielle Small
Kari Woldum
Elan Vital McAllister
Barbara Morningstar
Heather Struckman
Sophie Krupp
Maggie Hunter
Emilie Cellai Johnson
Rebekah Aliaghai
Angela Ashley Chiew
Bridget McGreevy
Lauren Brooks

Lainie Love Dalby
Alisa Blackwood
Linnea Bergvall
Nick Motter
Kitty Cavalier
Laura Farmer
Erin Niedermaier
Anne Ingman
Joanie Lamb
Christine Banas
Carlyn Shaw
Michael Fleres
Mahabisa Adam
Paul Ulrickson
Amanda Bacon Dwinell
Heidi Lynn Andersen
Ashley Brown
Rachel and Ryan Ohr
Katie Brooks
One Love Chiropractic (Asheville)
Andrea Ursel
Kristy Ryner
Caitlin Lang
Ben Miller
Emma Anderson
Matthias Pilz
Brigette Brink
Karen Friedman
Linda Gillen
Kendra Cunov
Julie Maree
Sonia Madera
Ambar Gingerelli

Keri Brusven
Megan Edgington

APPENDIX A: WISDOM OF BIRTH

The following are some themes and pearls of wisdom that may arise when women and men make meaning from their birth experiences:

• A deep respect, appreciation, and connection (perhaps even a sense of oneness) with all mothers, including our own lineage of women

• Profound self-confidence, self-trust, and self-awe

• The resiliency of the human spirit in how one faces and overcomes hardship

• Unconditional love in its immensity

• Faith that something larger is supporting and orchestrating everything

• Experiencing a deep and unshakable knowing; intuition

• Harmony and synchronicity of an event's unfolding

• Love, connection, and respect for the body and its creative capacity

• Deep trust in self, others, life

• Feeling completely supported by the seen and unseen

• Utter surrender

• Deep vulnerability

• Strength, courage, resolve

- Total and complete presence

- Self-advocacy

- Empowerment and pride

- Rebirth of the self (birth/death/rebirth; a phoenix process)

- Transformation

- Gratitude

- Direct access to and experience of the creative power of the universe

- The rise of past pains, presenting at birth as an opportunity to heal

JOURNAL ACTIVITY

What are the essential truths you've drawn from your experience of birth?

APPENDIX B: CHART OF BIRTH STORY LAYERS

Body Metaphor	Shared Qualities	Includes	Aspect of Being	Aspect of Story	Language Elements	Our Role	Key Elements
Skin Surface	outer layer covers protects continuity container for deeper structures	external landscape the facts when where what who timing + chronology	physical	setting context action	nouns verbs quantity the concrete	Actors: enact roles + reveal traits through behavior	starting point acceptable social story least vulnerable virtually unchange-able
Muscle Heart & Uterus	prime movers generate + coordinate action store + release energy strong + hardworking dynamic + changing	internal landscape thoughts feelings needs perception of events + relation-ships	emotional mental relational	character develop-ment mood	adjectives quality nuance	Agents: act upon inner desires, goals, values + plans	changeable shift from victimhood, shame + limiting beliefs change relationship to skin
Bones Soul	indestruc-tible what re-mains when all else falls away deep structure and form protects most vital holds us together	meaning why our stories matter lessons wisdom enduring truths	spiritual	themes morals messages	imagery symbol metaphor archetype	Authors: we take stock of life to craft story about who we've been, who we are, and who we are becoming	connection to collective experience themes and values integration + deep healing not revealed without reflection

APPENDIX C: THE BIRTH STORY GUIDE

This birth story guide is a helpful tool to find your way into your story and its details before crafting your narrative. It is meant to be as inclusive as possible, but not all questions will be relevant or resonant for all people. Please adapt this guide to make it your own.

Before Pregnancy

How did you feel about having children before this pregnancy? As a child? As an adult? Before and after you met your partner?

Did you and your partner plan this pregnancy? Was it a surprise?

What were your ideas/beliefs about pregnancy, birth, and parenthood before this journey began for you?

What were you told about your own birth and the other births in your family? What were you told about birth in general? How did these stories and ideas shape your own thoughts and feelings about pregnancy, birth, and motherhood?

Is this your first pregnancy? If not, what were the previous pregnancies like for you? How were your previous births? How did these experiences color your current birth experience?

Pregnancy

What was your experience around conception? Do you remember or have an idea of the time around which your baby was conceived? What is relevant about this time in your life? Was it easy or difficult to conceive? What else?

How did you discover you (or your partner) were pregnant? What were your first thoughts and feelings about the pregnancy? How did this change over time?

How did your partner feel/react to/support your pregnancy? In what ways is your relationship to the father/your partner relevant to your birth story?

In what memorable ways did others in your life react to news of your pregnancy (other children, parents, siblings, friends, relatives)?

If you have children already, what did you feel in relation to them while pregnant? How did you feel about bringing another child into your family?

What were your biggest fears surrounding birth?

What were your expectations about birth?

What were your hopes for birth?

What was your pregnancy like? What was your prenatal care like? Any particular care providers who stand out or who influenced you in a particular way?

How did you prepare yourself physically, emotionally, mentally, and spiritually for your birth and becoming a parent? Did you take any classes or read any books? How did they influence you?

Did you choose to know the sex of your baby? Why?

Did you select a name or names before baby's arrival? What was that process like?

Did you write a birth plan? What were your preferences and wishes? How did you share these with your care team, and how did you feel about their response to them?

What is relevant about your last months and weeks of pregnancy? How did you prepare yourself for birth then? How did you spend your time in anticipation of baby's arrival? What was your emotional experience of these last weeks and days before labor began?

Early Labor

I realized I was in labor at/around __:__ a.m./p.m. on ____ (day)
_____ (date) _____ (year) when _____
_____ (what happened). I was at
_____ doing _____
_____ (activity).

My _____ (partner, support person) was at
_____(location). S/he joined me (at/
when) _____.

I would describe my environment at this time as (season, weather, lighting, smells, sounds, temperature, etc.):

The people with me at the time included:

I would describe early labor as:

My contractions were (intensity, frequency, duration):

Physically, I felt:

Emotionally, I felt:

During early labor, I did the following/this happened (positions, comfort measures, distractions, events, interactions with others, location):

I found the following comforting/helpful:

What stands out/is notable about early labor?

How did your early labor compare to what you expected?

Active Labor

Active labor contractions began at/around __:__ a.m./p.m. on _____
(day) _____ (date) _____ (year). I could tell/I knew things were
changing because _____
_____, and I was at
_____ (location).

I would describe my environment at this time as (lighting, smells,
time of day, sounds, temperature, notable objects and individuals in
your environment):

The people with me at this time included:

I would describe active labor as:

My contractions were (intensity, frequency, duration):

Physically, I felt:

Emotionally, I felt:

During active labor, I did the following/this happened (positions, comfort measures, location changes, personal interactions, internal experiences, outer experiences):

I found the following comforting/helpful:

This is what stands out/is notable about this part of my labor (what you thought or experienced, what someone else did or said, etc.):

How did your active labor compare to what you expected?

What were the highs and lows of your active labor?

Transport (relevant if you moved from one location to another during your birth process)

I had to/decided to move from _____
(location 1) to _____ (location 2) when _____
_____ because _____
_____.

I would describe this experience as:

It affected my labor and/or overall birth experience in the following ways:

Interventions (if applicable)

The interventions/medical assistance we elected to have/needed were:

They happened at this time:

They changed my labor in the following ways:

Emotionally, I felt:

Physically, I felt:

What is noteworthy about this aspect of my birth experience is:

Transition

(This is the part of labor when a woman becomes fully dilated and moves from this phase of labor toward the pushing phase; many experience this part of labor as distinct from what came before and what comes after.)

What was transition like for you?

Did you know you were in transition? How did you know?

What thoughts were going through your head? What emotions did you feel?

What was happening around you at this time?

How did transition compare to what you had expected?

What helped you through transition?

Pushing/Birthing

I began to feel the urge or was told to push at/around __:__ a.m./ p.m. on _____ (day) _____ (date) _____ (year). I could tell/I knew things were changing because _____.
I was at _____(location).

I would describe my environment at this time as:

The people with me at this time included:

I would describe pushing as:

Physically, I felt:

Emotionally, I felt:

During the pushing/birthing stage, I did the following/this happened:

I found the following comforting/helpful:

This is what stands out about pushing/birthing my baby (what you thought, felt or experienced, what someone else did/said, etc.):

How did this stage of labor compare to what you expected?

Cesarean birth (if applicable)

I knew that I would be having a cesarean birth when:

The reason we opted for/needed a cesarean birth was:

I felt the following emotions about having a cesarean birth (before and now):

I would describe my birth as:

Physically, I felt:

Emotionally, I felt:

During the birth, I did the following/this happened:

I found the following comforting:

What stands out about the birth (what you thought or experienced, what someone else did or said, what surprised you):

What it comes to my cesarean birth, I am most happy/least happy about:

Birth

My baby was born at __:__ a.m./p.m. on _____ (day) _____ (date)
_____ (year) on/in _____
(where you delivered specifically—water, bed, floor, etc.) at _____
_____ (location) in _____
_____ (city, state).

The total length of my labor was _____ hours.

Physically, the birth of my baby felt like:

Emotionally, mentally, and spiritually, the birth of my baby felt like:

My first words after birth were:

During this time, my partner/support people did, said, etc.:

Baby was born _____ pounds _____ ounces and was _____ inches long.

My first impression or thoughts about my new baby were:

The first things that my baby did/that happened to my baby were:

Other notable things that happened in the moments before and short-ly after birth include:

After birth/placental stage

I began to birth my placenta around _____ minutes after birth. I was _____ (location). My baby was _____ (location).

I would describe this stage as:

What stands out about this stage is:

How did this stage of labor compare to what you'd expected?

Early hours/days with baby

After the birth, the following things happened (consider any aftercare you or baby needed; where baby, partner, and support people were; first experiences breastfeeding; baby's first exam; care team actions/conversations):

I would describe this time as:

The people with me at this time included:

Physically, I felt:

Emotionally, I felt:

My first experiences breastfeeding were:

What was significant about baby's first exam was:

What I ate after birth was:

What stands out in these early hours and days were:

Holding my baby during this time I felt:

Other things I remember about what happened after birth are:

Going home

We stayed at our place of birth for _____ (dura-tion). I was ready/not ready to go home at that point.

We returned home at/around __:__ a.m./p.m. on _____ (day) _____ (date) _____ (year).

I would describe my experience of going home as:

My baby was dressed in:

The car we drove home in was:

The weather was:

We live(d) in/at:

What stands out in the early hours and days at home with baby:

What was hard about the early days:

What was awesome about the early days:

The support I had in the early days:

The support I wish I'd had in the early days:

I would describe my recovery as:

I would describe my experiences getting to know my baby as:

Other thoughts about the birth and our first days and weeks at home
are:

Reflecting on your birth

The lowest point for me physically or emotionally during labor was:

The highest point for me physically or emotionally during labor was:

The thing that surprised me most about labor was:

This is how I felt about myself after birthing my baby:

I gained the following insight from my birth experience:

What I learned from my birth was:

If I could do it all over again, what I wish I'd known before labor was:

What I would do differently:

What I would do the same:

Given this experience, what I would want other women to know about birth is:

What I want my child to know about his/her birth is:

What my birth means to me on the deepest levels of my being:

What I believe about myself, others, or the world after this birth experience:

How my birth connects to the other parts of my life:

What has changed about my relationship to _____ is:

APPENDIX D: BIRTH STORY MEDITATION

This may be something you record and listen to before you write as a way to connect with the birth energy and your memory of birth. This meditation is also available on the website JaimeFleres.com for those who've purchased this book by using the following code: AUD123. With this meditation, you may want to close your eyes and just let your mind guide you in thought. You may also want to take notes during this meditation based on what comes up for you. It is entirely up to you. If something doesn't resonate or fit with your birth experience, let that be an opportunity for you to connect even more deeply with your own experience and follow that.

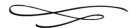

Let's first start by connecting with ourselves in the present moment. Notice your body, the beat of your heart, your breath. Settle your focus on your breath and take three deep breaths in through the nose and out through the mouth, sighing if needed. Fill up the lungs like you were filling up an accordion, expanding outwards toward your upper arms, and exhale, letting your ribs fall toward the midline of your body. Take a few more breaths like this, while slowing down and evening out the breath. Notice how you are feeling in your body right now. Where is there tension? Can you send your breath there and invite it to release?

Now settle your attention at your center, your core, your root, your womb—the place where you nurtured your baby and from which you birthed him or her. Imagine a big beautiful light emanating from this place and call forth the birth energy. Set an intention to remember all the details of your birth experience in the following moments in a way that will prepare you to write. Honor yourself for the tremendous effort you devoted to carrying and birthing your baby.

Let's begin at the beginning of your story. Where is that for you? When does your birth story begin? It can begin wherever you like. Does it begin with your own birth? Your childhood? Sometime in your adulthood? Does it begin with the last time you gave birth? With your conception of this pregnancy? During pregnancy? Or perhaps it begins during the labor itself? What comes first?

As you move through this beginning, come to your conception.
What was this experience like for you?
Was it easy? Difficult?
How did you find out you were pregnant?
How did you feel? How did you share the news?
What was going on in your life at the time?
What was your pregnancy like?
Are there moments or parts of the pregnancy that really stand out?
What was your prenatal care like?
What else about your pregnancy is relevant to your birth story?
How did you feel in the last weeks of your pregnancy as you prepared for baby's arrival?
As you are ready, move to the time when you knew that labor was beginning.
Where are you? Is it day or night? Who are you with? What is the weather like outside?
What happens during this time? What is this experience like for you?
What rhythms, rituals, and comforts of birth are working for you?
What else is going on during your early labor?
Follow your story through to the first major shift.
What changes here? Do you move into active labor?
Do you move from one place to another?
Does day become night or night become day?
Something else?
What is this shift like?
How does it feel?

Continue on through this part of your story. Follow it through your labor, whatever this looked like for you.

What was the rest of your labor like?

What stands out?

What do you remember about your inner experience as you moved through the birth process?

What do you remember about your surroundings—the place where you birth and the people who are there?

What else arises about this time in your birth experience?

Follow this memory until the time just before you meet your baby.

You are about to meet your baby for the first time. You've carried this baby so well for many, many months, and you've made a tremendous effort throughout your labor. Maybe you have been pushing hard, and you can feel baby crowning. Maybe you are in surgery and you know that you'll be meeting your baby soon.

Where are you?

How are you feeling?

What thoughts are running through your mind?

What else is alive for you now?

Go to the time when your baby is being born and the moments immediately after.

What are you thinking and feeling at this time?

What do you remember about when you first saw and held your baby?

What is your partner's initial reaction? Others in the room?

Do you remember anything you or someone else said at this time?

What else is going on around you at this time?

Now connect to the hours after baby was born.

What was significant about this time?

Did you breastfeed? What was that like?

Did your baby get his or her first exam? What do you remember from that?

What was your first meal after birth?

What thoughts and feelings came up for you during these early hours with your new baby?

Connect now with your overall experience of this birth.

What were the highs and lows for you during this birth experience?

How did you feel about yourself after giving birth?

What insight did you gain as a result of your birth experience?

What did you learn from this birth?

In what ways did birth affect you emotionally, mentally, spiritually?

Now follow the narrative in your mind to the end of your story. Where does your birth story end? Just like the beginning, it can end wherever you like. Perhaps it ends when baby arrives? Or when you leave your birth place? Or during the postpartum as you reflect on the birth and being a mother? Does it end with some insight you gained from this experience? Does it continue on to the next time you birth? Or to another event?

Take whatever time you need to come back to the room, but stay with your birth story and this birth energy. It is now time to express this narrative in written form. I encourage you to just start writing and let the thoughts and memories in your mind flow.

If you need further help getting started, please refer to Chapters 12 and 13.

APPENDIX E: QOYA-BASED MOVEMENT RITUAL

This is a movement ritual to assist you in connecting back with the energy of your birth experience as a way to prepare to write your story. Use this ritual before writing or anytime you wish to connect with and honor your experience.

Song One: CONNECT TO THE BIRTH ENERGY.

Lie on the floor with your hands at your sides or on your low belly. Close your eyes and slow your breath, moving into a balanced 4:4 breath pattern (four-count inhale, four-count exhale) and expanding this to a 6:6 or even an 8:8 breath. (You may also wish to use an alternate nostril breathing technique if this is familiar to you.) Begin to focus your inhales and exhales on your low belly, breathing into and out of the womb. Imagine a glowing light there that gets brighter on the inhale and expands on the exhale. During this time, if appropriate for your body, draw your belly button to your spine on the exhale and release completely on the inhale, repeating for the last minute of the song. (Feel free to extend this process to the length of two songs.) Intentionally call in the energy of your birth and become aware of its presence and your connection to it. Notice its quality, its feeling in your body. Witness and remain aware of all that arises in your body, heart, mind, and soul.

Song suggestions
"1/1 – 2004 Digital Remaster" by Brian Eno
"Priya (beloved)" by Benjy Wertheimer
"TwentyTwoFourteen" by The Album Leaf
"Faith's Hymn" by Beautiful Chorus
"Green Arrow" by Yo La Tengo

"Center" or "Savasana" by Josh Brill
"Devi Prayer" by Craig Pruess & Ananda (for a longer song choice)

Song Two: SHAKE OUT THE BLOCKS.

At your pace, stand and get ready to move! Put on an upbeat song and begin to systematically shake through each part of your body, focusing on each part for about twenty seconds. Begin with right foot, then left; shuffle both legs up and down like a football player; shake your tail like a happy puppy. Then shake your core (very gently or not at all if you're newly postpartum), shake your heart, shake your shoulders, your arms, your hands, all the way to your fingers. Then go back and shake whatever needs more shaking. Shake out any blocks or limits to your confidence and motivation to write your story. Give those worries, cares, and limitations to the earth. Shake out all that stands between you and the truth of your story.

Song suggestions
"Love Is Queen Omega" by Zuco 103
"Inni Mer Syngur Vitleysingur" by Sigur Rós
"Tamacun" by Rodrigo y Gabriela
"Shake It Out" by Florence + the Machine
"Shake It" by Michael Franti and Spearhead
"Wings" by Little Mix - DNA

Song Three: DANCE YOUR STORY.

Put on a song and dance your birth story. Don't let your mind dictate how you'll move; allow it to be a witness. Let your body tell the story of your birth. After all, the actual experience of birth happened in your body, and then your mind came in to make it a story. Allow the wisdom of your body to inform your story and connect fully to your birth experience.

Song suggestions
"True to Myself" by Ziggy Marley
"Brave" by Sara Bareilles
"Say" by John Mayer
"You Were Born" by Cloud Cult
"Life Is Better with You" by Michael Franti and Spearhead
"How Long Will I Love You" by Ellie Goulding

When you have finished this movement ritual, jot down anything you discovered in this process that you want to integrate into your written account or just start writing!

APPENDIX F: USING NVC TO PROCESS BIRTH TRAUMA IN WRITING

Nonviolent Communication (NVC), also known as Compassionate Communication or Collaborative Communication, is a communication process and philosophy developed by American psychologist Marshall Rosenberg in the 1960s. One of the major facets of NVC is developing and practicing self-empathy, which is defined as a deep and compassionate awareness of one's own inner experience.

NVC holds central the feelings and needs we each have in every moment and aspect of our lives; such needs and feelings are universal to all humans. Understanding our feelings and needs, both during our experience of birth and later as we process our experience, can be a tremendous asset as we seek to heal birth trauma through writing. We can take some of the more potent or troubling aspects of our experience, slow them down, and inspect them through NVC to gain more self-empathy and, hopefully, healing.

In classic NVC, there is a four-part process we can work through to gain greater self-awareness and greater self-empathy. (Please note: for the purposes of this book, I have greatly simplified this process, but to learn more I invite you to read some of the recommended texts listed at the end of the book.) This four-part process includes:

- Making a neutral observation about what happened;
- Describing the feeling(s) we had and have in relation to that occurrence;
- Identifying the needs we had/have that were met or unmet in relation to that experience; and
- Making a request of ourselves or someone else.

Let's go through an example from one woman's experience of birth.

Observation

During my cesarean birth, I could hear the doctor talking and joking with his colleagues about the big football game starting later that day.

This is just what happened, no layering of judgments or evaluations of it. We can have the version where we say, "That doctor was a total &$@!? and didn't even care about me or my birth!" but NVC invites us to strip our story of the interpretations, evaluations, and conclusions just long enough to open the possibility for new insights and processing to occur. It gets us off the well-worn paths our stories often tread.

Feelings then and now

When this happened, I felt humiliated and invisible. Today I feel angry and disappointed when I think about it.

Our feelings are ours. We work toward recognizing, understanding, and taking responsibility for them. This is not to heave more burden on our backs, but to take back ownership of our lives and our internal landscape. It is okay to feel exactly how we feel—and to allow the possibility of shifting and movement within our emotional landscape.

Needs then and now

When the doctor made small talk during my birth, my needs for acknowledgment, respect, consideration, and understanding were not met. My needs to be seen and to matter were not met, either. They still feel unmet.

Here, we have this great opportunity for self-empathy. We can look at what happened, how we felt and feel about it, and what we needed and now need. We can play the "how human of me" game, a favorite of my teacher Judith Lasater, author, NVC practitioner, and renowned yoga teacher. "How human of me to need to be acknowledged, respected, and given consideration during the birth of my child! How human of me to feel humiliated and angry when those needs were not met!" Here, we start to love ourselves just as we are, just as we were during our birth experience. We understand that our feelings and needs are normal and wonderful. It starts to make sense; we can bring more empathy and acceptance to our reactions and experiences.

Request

In the process of self-empathy, this step may be an internal exploration that may or may not involve outward action. How can we get our needs met in the present moment? Do we need to go back to the original situation? In our example, can she go back to the doctor and talk about the impact of his behavior on her birth experience? Is that what she needs? Can she meet those needs in another context? For example, could she share her story with another and ask if they are willing to meet her needs, i.e., to see, respect, and understand her? Alternatively, is it more appropriate that she acknowledge her unmet needs (allowing them the space to just be), grieve them, and give herself empathy and compassion through internal processes such as writing, movement, and internal dialogue?

Your Turn

STEP 1: OBSERVATION - Take a moment or aspect of your birth and state in neutral language what happened.

STEP 2: FEELINGS - Write about (1) your feelings connected to this event and (2) your feelings about this situation today. Here is a partial list to help you accurately name your feelings. (Feel free to use those not on the lists.)

Feelings When Our Needs Are Not Met

AFRAID
Apprehensive
Frightened
Mistrustful
Panicked
Scared
Fearful
Terrified

ANGRY
Enraged
Furious
Irate
Outraged
Uneasy
Unnerved
Unsettled
Upset

ANNOYED
Aggravated
Dismayed
Disgruntled
Exasperated
Frustrated
Impatient
Irritated

AVERSE
Appalled
Disgusted
Hateful
Horrified
Hostile
Repulsed

CONFUSED
Ambivalent
Baffled
Bewildered
Dazed
Hesitant
Lost
Mystified
Unsure

DEPRESSED
Dejected
Despairing
Despondent
Disappointed
Discouraged
Gloomy
Heavy-hearted
Hopeless
Sad
Unhappy
Weepy

DISCONNECTED
Apathetic
Cold
Detached
Distant
Distracted
Indifferent
Numb
Removed
Separated
Shut down
Withdrawn

DISTURBED
Agitated
Alarmed
Discombobulated
Rattled
Restless
Shocked
Startled
Surprised
Troubled

EMBARRASSED
Ashamed
Flustered
Humiliated
Guilty
Mortified
Self-Conscious

FATIGUED
Burnt Out
Depleted
Exhausted
Lethargic
Weary
Worn out

PAINED
Anguished
Bereaved
Grief
Heart-broken
Hurt
In agony
Lonely
Miserable
Regretful
Remorseful

ANXIOUS
Tense
Cranky
Distressed
Distraught
Edgy
Frazzled
Irritable
Overwhelmed
Restless

VULNERABLE
Fragile
Guarded
Helpless
Leery
Reserved
Sensitive
Shaky
Uncomfortable
Exposed

YEARNING
Envious
Jealous
Longing
Nostalgic

Feelings When Our Needs Are Met

AFFECTIONATE
Compassionate
Friendly
Loving
Open-hearted
Sympathetic
Tender
Warm

CONFIDENT
Empowered
Open
Proud
Safe
Secure

ENGAGED
Alert
Curious
Enchanted
Fascinated
Interested
Involved

EXCITED	GRATEFUL	CONTENT
Amazed	Appreciative	Calm
Astonished	Moved	Centered
Eager	Thankful	Clear-headed
Energetic	Touched	Comfortable
Enthusiastic		Fulfilled
Invigorated	HOPEFUL	Peaceful
Passionate	Encouraged	Quiet
Surprised	Optimistic	Relaxed
Vibrant		Relieved
	INSPIRED	Satisfied
EXHILARATED	Awed	Serene
Blissful	Amazed	Trusting
Ecstatic	In wonder	Whole
Pleased		
Radiant	JOYFUL	REFRESHED
Thrilled	Amused	Rejuvenated
	Delighted	Rested
	Glad	Restored
	Happy	Revived
	Pleased	

STEP 3: NEEDS - Identify the needs that were met or not met during this experience. Next, identify the need(s) you have now related to this experience. (This may offer you an indication of what actions you may wish to take now.) Here are the universal rights (we may call them needs) of all birthing women, according to the World Health Organization:

- Freedom from harm and ill-treatment
- Access to information
- Informed consent and refusal

- Respect for one's choices and preferences, including companionship during care
- Dignity and respect throughout care
- Equality; freedom from discrimination; equitable care
- Timely health care and the highest attainable level of care
- Liberty, autonomy, self-determination, and freedom from coercion

---

Universal Human Needs

BASIC	COMMUNITY & SUPPORT	OTHERS
Food	To belong	Ease
Water	To matter	Celebration
Air	To be heard	Mourning
Shelter	Acknowledgment	Presence
Health/Healing	Appreciation	Meaning
Sleep/Rest	Cooperation	Purpose
	Worth	Beauty
SAFETY		Wholeness
Order		Flow
Security	AUTONOMY	Courage
Fairness	Agency	Competence
Consideration	Choice	Contribution
Protection	Control	Responsibility
Familiarity	Freedom	Reliability
Privacy	Self-efficacy	
	Power	
EMPATHY	Space	
Respect	Independence	
Understanding	Integrity	
Acceptance	Clarity	
Connection	Openness	
Love	Self-expression	

STEP 4: REQUEST - What do you want to do with the information you have just gathered? Do you need acknowledgment and self-empathy? Can you offer yourself what you needed then/need now through a written or internal dialogue process? Would you like to request that someone else witness your story and help meet your needs (or find a way to meet them)? Do you need to return to the original situation?

Optional Exercise: Turning It Around

Sometimes we heal by extending our empathy to others in a difficult situation. This can be a tough and brave thing to do. We may not want to empathize with that insensitive "jock doc" (not an NVC label, by the way), but we might want to consider the following turn-around: Go through the same process but imagine you are in the doctor's shoes. Imagine what he was feeling and needing in the situation as a way to see him as a human who was also trying to get his needs met. (Apply this turning-around practice to your own experience, of course.)

This process is in no way meant to justify mistreatment or mistakes. This isn't a gift to them; it is a gift to ourselves. In this process, we develop the ability to offer others empathy (another major facet of the NVC process). We do this to find peace for ourselves.

APPENDIX G: ADDITIONAL WRITING PROMPTS

After you have completed a narrative form of your birth story, you may want to alter genres and see what wisdom and insight this new form yields. Alternatively, if the basic storytelling motif doesn't suit you, you might wish to write a less conventional birth story—and some of the ideas below may appeal to you. Lastly, there are healing gems to be gleaned from writing in one of the following ways.

Prompt 1: Shift Perspective

Write the story from a different perspective—your baby/child, partner, relative, care provider, an extraterrestrial. What does your birth look like from this vantage? What new insights surface when looking at your birth through another's imagined perspective?

Prompt 2: Write in Third Person

Write your story in third person. Instead of saying *I*, *me*, and *my*, use *she* and *her*. Notice what effect this has on your storytelling. Does it lend you more breathing room between you and the story? Do you discover something new about the story you didn't see before? More self-compassion?

Prompt 3: Write about a Single Moment

Take the most powerful moment of your story and write only about it. Focus on this moment and extract from it all the sensory details, all the internal details, all that you can. Explore it from every angle. What happened? What did it mean?

Prompt 4: Write a Letter to Heal

Write a letter to a care provider or someone involved in your birth to express your emotions or as a way to get a specific angle in your writing that produces a distinct version of your story. This can be incredibly healing if you have difficult or unresolved emotions toward someone who was (or wasn't) present at your birth. Maybe your partner missed the birth, and while you understand, you need a space to process your disappointment and grief. Maybe you write a letter to a child you have lost or to a parent who has passed. Perhaps your care provider was insensitive and did not support you in the way you needed—you can write a letter to them and say everything you need to say. Whether you ever show it to them is irrelevant to your healing journey.

Forgiveness experts report that great healing comes when we imagine the person we need to forgive is sitting in front of us, and we tell them everything we need to say. And remember, forgiveness is a gift you give to yourself, not to another. You don't need their participation to get closure and a sense of resolution in the aftermath of a trauma or hurt. You may also decide to share your feelings with this other person, and your writing can be a vehicle for this expression.

Prompt 5: Write a Letter of Gratitude

On the other hand, your letter to a person connected to your birth might be one of celebration and great gratitude. You might use this form to give thanks, to recognize someone who supported you, to honor their role in the birth, and to use writing as a way of both expressing and remembering this sentiment.

Prompt 6: Write a Letter to Past or Future You

Write a letter to yourself—either "past you" or "future you" about your birth experience. If writing to "past you," tell her what you discovered in your birthing experience, what you wished she knew then that you know now. If writing to "future you," what do you want to remind her about, something that is clear to you now?

Prompt 7: Write a Poem

The creativity that comes from poetic form may be a liberating or natural way for you to express your experience of birth. It might be a way to get at those deeper, rich truths about your birth experience that may not be otherwise possible in a different writing form. Poetry, a short poem perhaps, may be less intimidating than writing a long narrative prose piece.

I have included the birth poem I wrote (see page 160). Of course, this is just one example. Perhaps you start with a central image that you connect to your story—the breath, a cry, some tangible item that holds meaning for your experience, a sound, a smell, an image, a taste, or one of the birth "truths" listed in Appendix A.

Prompt 8: The Three-Card Birth Story

This is a writing exercise that comes from the Qoya practice.

• If you have oracle cards, choose a deck, two, or three, and spread them out face down in front of you.

• Invite your intuition to select three cards, determining which will be card 1, card 2, and card 3. Keep them face down in front of you. Card 1 will inform the beginning of your story, card 2 the middle, and card 3 the end of your story.

• Take out your journal and write the most relevant of these sentences: "Once upon a time, there was a woman who gave birth to a child..." or "Once upon a time, there was a (wo)man who witnessed the birth of a child..." This is a stream-of-consciousness kind of writing exercise, so try not to overthink it. Just go where your mind-heart-spirit leads you.

• Flip the first card and use the words or images on the card to begin writing the beginning of your story. Write in the third person for ten minutes.

• Next, flip the second card and write the middle of your story for the next ten minutes.

• Then, flip the third card and take ten minutes to write the ending of your story.

• When you are done, read through your story exactly as it is. Notice the effects of reading this story in the third person.

• Next, go through and change all the third-person pronouns to the first person. Now it becomes "Once upon a time, I was a woman who gave birth to my child," and so on. Where it says *she*, change to *I*; where it says *her*, change to *me* or *my*.

• Read your story again in the first person and notice its effects.

• Reflect on what themes and ideas emerged from this practice.

Prompt 9: Write Your Birth Story in Fifty Words or Less

This can help you capture only what is most essential to your story. If you are anything like me, you may try to squeeze every detail of your memories into the bucket of your birth story. This has great benefits, but so does brevity. Give yourself the challenge (or gift) of writing only fifty words or so about the birth. Distill what is truly essential and write that. This doesn't mean whittling it down to a list of "facts," but maybe it will give you permission to write what birth was really about for you. Maybe it won't have any of those practical facts at all but will reveal the essence of your experience.

Prompt 10: Write and Burn

Write about the dark, gritty parts of your story that you are too afraid to write—the parts you've been suppressing, holding back, keeping in the shadows. The parts you don't want anyone to see (maybe even yourself!). Give yourself permission to write the brutal truth. Give your anger, your hurt, your disappointment, or your grief full creative license to let loose. Give yourself the reassurance that this work will never see much light of day. When you are done writing whatever needs to be expressed, burn your writing. Let this be a ritual to move this energy and release the burdens of having to carry all of this alone. Offer it up to something greater for transmutation. When we are not actively using our energy to suppress negative emotions, we clear our energy up for other things!

Prompt 11: Think beyond the Birth Story

While outside the scope of "birth story writing," I encourage you to also tell stories about your life as a parent beyond the birthing experience. Write a story about your pregnancy, about your postpartum period, about nursing, about weaning, about your child as a baby, about a funny or memorable event in your family life. Tell your stories! And keep on telling them.

NOTES

Part One: Why Write?

1. Dederer, Claire. "Not Telling." In *Labor Day: True Birth Stories by Today's Best Women Writers*, edited by Henderson, Eleanor and Anna Solomon, 283. New York: Farrar, Straus, and Giroux, 2014.

2. Bonheim, Jalaja. *Aphrodite's Daughters: Women's Sexual Stories and the Journey of the Soul*. New York: Simon & Schuster, 1997, 259.

3. Simkin, Penny. "Just Another Day in a Woman's Life? Women's Long-Term Perceptions of Their First Birth Experience." *Birth* 18, no. 4 (December 1991): 203–210.

4. Greenberg, Arielle. "The Tigers in the Room." In *Labor Day: True Birth Stories by Today's Best Women Writers*, edited by Henderson, Eleanor and Anna Solomon, 252. New York: Farrar, Straus, and Giroux, 2014.

5. Keane, Mary Beth. "Weight." In *Labor Day: True Birth Stories by Today's Best Women Writers*, edited by Henderson, Eleanor and Anna Solomon, 215. New York: Farrar, Straus, and Giroux, 2014.

6. Harris, Judith. *Signifying Pain: Construction and Healing the Self through Writing*. Albany: State University of New York Press, 2003.

7. Beck, Cheryl Tatano. "Post-Traumatic Stress Disorder Due to Childbirth." *Nursing Research* 53, no. 4 (July/August 2004): 216–225.

8. Webster, Rachel Jamison. "The Broken." In *Labor Day: True Birth Stories by Today's Best Women Writers*, edited by Henderson, Eleanor and Anna Solomon, 128-129. New York: Farrar, Straus, and Giroux, 2014.

9. Panuthos, Claudia. *Transformation through Birth: A Woman's Guide*. New York: Bergin & Garvey, 1984, 37.

10. Houser, Patrick. "The Science of Father Love." n.d. http://birthpsychology.com/free-article/science-father-love (accessed October 2015).

11. Kaitz, M., Shiri, S., Danzinger, S. et al. "Fathers can also recognize their children by touch." *Infant Behaviour and Development* 17 (1984): 205-07.

Works Consulted

Beck, Cheryl Tatano. "Pentatic Cartography: Mapping Birth Trauma Narratives." *Qualitative Health Research* 16, no. 4 (April 2006): 453-466.

Pennebaker, James and Joshua Smyth. *Opening Up by Writing It Down: How Expressive Writing Improves Health and Eases Emotional Pain*. New York: Guilford Press, 2016.

Odent, Michel. "Is the Participation of the Father at Birth Dangerous?" *Midwifery Today*, Autumn 1999.

Part Two: Anatomy of a Birth Story

1. "Brené Brown: How Vulnerability Can Make Our Lives Better." https://www.forbes.com/sites/danschawbel/2013/04/21/brene-brown-how-vulnerability-can-make-our-lives-better/#554c945936c7 Accessed 19 August 2017.

2. Estés, Clarissa Pinkola. *Women Who Run with the Wolves: Myths and Stories of the Wild Woman Archetype*. New York: Ballentine, 1995, p. 33.

3. Greer, Carl. *Change Your Story, Change Your Life: Using Shamanic and Jungian Tools to Achieve Personal Transformation*. Scotland: Findhorn Press, 2014.

Works Consulted

Beck, Julie. *Story of My Life: How Narrative Creates Personality*. August 10, 2015. http://www.theatlantic.com/heath/archive/2015/08/life-stories-narrative-psychology-redemption-mental-health/400796/ (accessed September 11, 2015).

England, Pam. *BHJ Continued: Story Gate Three: Relationships*. n.d. http://birthpeeps.blogspot.com/2011/07/bhj-continued-story-gate-three.html (accessed September 26, 2016).

Part Three: How to Write

Works Consulted

DeSalvo, Louise. *Writing as a Way of Healing: How Telling Our Stories Transforms Our Lives*. Boston: Beacon Press, 1999.

Goldberg, Natalie. *Writing Down the Bones: Freeing the Writer Within*. Boston: Shambhala, 2005.

Lamott, Ann. *Bird by Bird: Some Instructions on Writing and Life*. Anchor Books, 1995.

RESOURCES

These are just a few of my very favorite books on these topics.

Books

Birth Story Anthologies

Mann, Jennifer Derryberry, ed. *Belly Button Bliss: A Small Collection of Happy Birth Stories*. Minneapolis: Fairview Press, 2010.

Henderson, Eleanor and Anna Solomon, ed. *Labor Day: True Birth Stories by Today's Best Women Writers*. New York: Farrar, Straus, and Giroux, 2014.

Books about Birth and Parenthood

Dick-Read, Grantly and Ina May Gaskin. *Childbirth Without Fear: Principles and Practice of Natural Childbirth*. London: Pinter and Martin, 2013.

England, Pam and Rob Horowitz. *Birthing from Within*. Albuquerque: Partera Press, 1998.

Gaskin, Ina May. *Spiritual Midwifery*. Summertown: Book Publishing Company, 2002.

---. *Ina May's Guide to Childbirth*. New York: Bantam, 2003.

Kent, Tami Lynn. *Mothering from Your Center: Tapping Your Body's Natural Energy for Pregnancy, Birth, and Parenting*. New York: Atria Books, 2013.

Romm, Aviva. *The Natural Pregnancy Book* (1997), *Natural Health after Birth: The Complete Guide to Postpartum Wellness* (2002), *Naturally Healthy Babies and Children* (2000), and more

St. John, Rose. *Fathers at Birth: Your Role in Bringing Your Child into the World*. Portland: Ringing Bell Press, 2009.

Wright Glenn, Amy. *Birth, Breath and Death: Meditations on Motherhood, Chaplaincy, and Life as a Doula*. CreateSpace, 2013.

Nonviolent Communication Books

Rosenberg, Marshall. *Nonviolent Communication: A Language of Life*, 2nd ed. Encinitas: Puddle Dancer Press, 2003.

Lasater, Judith. *What We Say Matters: Practicing Non-Violent Communication*. Berkeley: Rodmell Press, 2009.

Other Relevant Books/Authors

Brown, Brené. –Any of her works.

Hopper, Kate. *Use Your Words: A Writing Guide for Mothers*. Berkeley: Viva, 2012.

Katie, Byron and Stephen Mitchell. *Loving What Is: Four Questions That Can Change Your Life*. New York: Harmony Books, 2002.

Schieck, Rochelle. *Qoya: A Compass for Navigating an Embodied Life That Is Wise, Wild, and Free*. New York: Inspire and Move, 2016.

Van Der Kolk, Bessel. *The Body Keeps the Score: Brain, Mind, and Body in the Healing of Trauma*. New York: Penguin, 2014.

Online and Professional Resources

Pregnancy Support after Loss

https://pregnancyafterlosssupport.com/

Birth Story Medicine

birthingfromwithin.com/pages/birth-story-medicine

Birth Art Sessions

bfwclasses.com

Core Belief support

Susan Shehata offers Core Story work to help us release the beliefs that hold us back from the life we desire. SusanShehata.com/StoryWork

LiYana Silver, a women's coach and author who also supports working through limiting core beliefs. LiyanaSilver.com

ABOUT THE AUTHOR

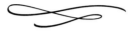

Born and raised in the San Francisco Bay Area, Jaime Fleres (Mizejewski) has been writing to process, heal, and honor her life experiences since she was an early teenager. She received her bachelor's degree in Women's Studies and English (Summa Cum Laude) and her master's degree in the Teaching of Writing from San Diego State University. She enjoyed several years as a composition and literature professor both in California and Minnesota. After giving birth to her daughter in 2013, she founded a holistic birth and wellness business, Santosha Birth and Wellness, became a doula and certified to teach both yoga and Qoya. She offers private writing guidance, workshops, and retreats for men and women about writing the stories that matter. Jaime currently lives in Asheville, North Carolina with her husband, daughter, two dogs, and cat. Learn more about Jaime at JaimeFleres.com.

Made in United States
North Haven, CT
05 July 2022

20944576R00190